EDUCATION AND PREVENTIVE MEDICINE

COLUMBIA
UNIVERSITY PRESS
SALES AGENTS
NEW YORK:
LEMCKE & BUECHNER
30–32 WEST 27TH STREET

LONDON:
HENRY FROWDE
AMEN CORNER, E.C.

EDUCATION AND PREVENTIVE MEDICINE

BY

NORMAN EDWARD DITMAN, Ph.D., M.D.

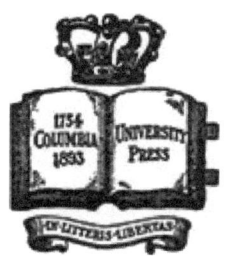

New York
THE COLUMBIA UNIVERSITY PRESS
1911
All rights reserved

This paper originally appeared in June, 1908, as a supplement to Volume X, Number 3, of the COLUMBIA UNIVERSITY QUARTERLY, under the title: "Education and its Economic Value in the Field of Preventive Medicine. The Need of a School of Sanitary Science and Public Health." It has been for a long time out of print. Constant demands for it, from many parts of the country, have led to this second printing by the Columbia University Press.

EDUCATION AND PREVENTIVE MEDICINE

Great as has been the progress of civilization since the early centuries, the greatest advances have occurred during the cycle just completed. Exceeding all other periods of time in the marvelous development of the sciences and arts, the nineteenth century stands for achievements of which the human race may well be proud. But great as was the material, intellectual, and social progress of **Greatest advance of the 19th century** the world during the past century, there is no advance which compares, in its influence upon the happiness of mankind, with the increased power to lessen physical suffering from disease and accident and to control the spread of pestilence.

The dangers arising from the spread of contagious and other infectious diseases threaten, not the individual only, but the industrial life and the whole fabric of modern society. **An enormous amount of disease still exists** While our progress in the power to conquer disease has been great, there is a growing tendency to allow the glory of past achievement to obscure the magnitude of the field of tasks still undone. Reforms and the adoption of new methods, while accomplishing much, have had a tendency to stimulate our efforts in directions where the greatest returns are not secured from the degree of effort invested.

In all attempts to remove great evils it is the dictate of wisdom to select those agencies which are most likely to bring about the **Removal of evil by destruction of its root** greatest results with the least labor or sacrifice of means. Since time began it has been an economic axiom that the most effective manner of accomplishing this result is by nipping the evil in the bud, or digging up and destroying the roots, rather than by lopping off only its branches. A great amount of time, labor, and money are consumed in dealing with the *effects* of evils, without reducing or removing their chief sources or primary causes. Thus, in the history of diseases, while there has been an immense expenditure of labor and means to *cure* these evils, comparatively little has been

Past failure to apply this principle done to *prevent* them. The same holds true with respect to crime, pauperism, and insanity. Disease, crime, pauperism, insanity, and preventable accidents, are the foulest blots on the modern civilized state, and the responsibility for the amelioration of these curses must be faced, upon the last analysis, by the medical profession. But the education of the physician in the past, while fitting him for the overcoming of isolated problems, has absolutely lacked that comprehensiveness needed to enable him to obtain a mastery of the broader economic and social problems of our modern life. For example, such a man should not only be able to cure, but should understand the problems of the prevention of disease and the investigation of its causes; he should be familiar with the methods of public health administration involving the health of the city, the State, and the country, which bear upon the purity of food and water supplies, the existence of dangerous occupations, and the occurrence of epidemics. He should be a master of sociological questions involving the habits of the people and the evils of tenement house existence. He should be familiar with methods of municipal finance and government, questions of commerce, economics, and medical jurisprudence. He should be conversant with the mental, moral, and physical aspects of educational questions, direct the labors of charitable organizations and social workers, and educate the public through personal contract, the press, the school, and the higher institutions of learning.

The need of such men is at once apparent, and while the fact **Reason for this failure** has, up to the present, been little appreciated, it is painfully true that nowhere in this broad land is there any place where such training may be obtained.

Only a few years ago our inaccurate knowledge of the cause of disease made sanitation a blundering science; but the knowledge, **Promise of relief** recently acquired, of the causation and modes of spreading of disease, and of methods of acquiring immunity, has transformed the face of modern medicine, and the boon of supreme import to the human race has been the lesson that most diseases are preventable.

Pasteur has truthfully said: "It is within the power of man to make all infectious diseases disappear from the world." How

Possible to prevent disease appalling, then, are the ravages of disease, when we consider that of the 1,000,000 deaths annually in this country of 76,000,000 people, 40 per cent. or 400,000 are unnecessary, and with our present knowledge of their cause can be prevented. Eleven hundred deaths every day as a sacrifice to the ignorance, carelessness, and inertia of the multitude!

Of the human beings born alive in this civilized country more than one-third die before the age of five years has been attained.
Great sacrifice of children 307,562 deaths out of 875,521, coming within this class (1). The sum of sorrow to the living, and the loss to the ranks of the world's producers which these statements represent are deplorable.

But perhaps the most astonishing impression follows from the consideration of the economic loss to the country which these figures **Great economic loss** represent. Hunter (2) has estimated the average cost of preparing a man for usefulness at $1,500. This is in the nature of a grant from parents or the state which the child, when he becomes a man, is expected to return to the community by his labor. The loss of 400,000 workers from preventable disease, therefore, represents an annual loss to the country of $600,000,000.

A striking example of the economic gain which results from the saving of human life is the following: England reckons that the lives saved through the lowered death-rate, from what it was between 1866 and 1875, to what it became in the period reaching from 1880 to 1889, amounted to 858,804 (3). This represents on the English basis of the per capita valuation of each life ($770), a social capital of $650,000,000 saved ($1,285,206,000 on the basis of Hunter's estimate). In ten years England has more than regained the sum spent in fifteen years for sanitary improvements, though the average annual expenditure has been $42,000,000.

In New York City, the decrease in the death-rate resulting from methods of prevention, for twenty-five years of 5.89 per 1,000 **Economic saving of preventive measures in New York** inhabitants, represents a saving of over 3,500 lives annually, and of over 80,000 lives during the quarter of a century (3). The social capital saved—using Hunter's valuation—amounts to

$120,000,000. Adding further to this the reduced number of sick cases, usually reckoned as twenty-eight to each death, the average duration of illness at nine days, and the daily wage at $1.50, the total saving to society exclusive of nursing, medicines, etc., reaches the sum of $150,240,000. This reduction of sickness and death saved the work of three great hospitals; it saved many wives from being widows and many children from being fatherless; and it also saved many from poverty. This is the work of prevention. The same saving should be made again and again. This year, if perfect sanitary measures could be put into effect, probably 20,000 or 25,000 lives could be saved in New York City alone, and 200,000 cases of severe illness prevented.

An added gain from the principles of prevention results from the increased average length of life, which has risen from $21\frac{1}{4}$ years in the sixteenth century to $40\frac{1}{2}$ years in the nineteenth century: certainly a brilliant result (4).

Increased span of life

The assurance of the continued advance in the beneficial results of preventive medicine in the future is confirmed by a survey of its steady triumphs in the past, and it is only by a comparison of the depths of misery and suffering of past centuries, with our latter-day comparative freedom from disease with the guarantee of continued progress in this line that the true importance of methods of prevention is appreciated.

The horrors of epidemic pestilence and the part played by modern science in overcoming it, are very typically exemplified by the history of the bubonic plague or Black Death. This disease has ravaged Africa, Asia, and Europe almost from time immemorial. It is said that Athens once lost more than one-third of its population by such an epidemic, and the great plague reported by Livy is said to have destroyed a million persons in Africa during the third century before Christ. In England, in 1348, it spread with such terrible rapidity that within a few months almost every town and village throughout the country had been attacked, and in some places only a fourth part of the inhabitants were left alive. In London alone 100,000 fell victims to the disease, and 50,000

Losses by disease in past centuries

Destruction due to the plague

corpses were interred in one burial-ground, heaped together, layer upon layer, in large pits. Throughout Europe it has been estimated that twenty-five millions, or a fourth part of the entire population, were swept away. Imagination fails to realize the misery and horrors of the time—everywhere there was terror and despair. In the seventeenth century 400,000 were destroyed, and in the eighteenth century 250,000 fell a prey to this scourge. During the nineteenth century there were few years when small epidemics were not active in some region of what is known as the "plague belt" (5).

While comparatively isolated outbreaks of plague have occurred in Asiatic countries from time to time in later years, it seemed improbable that there would be any more extensive epidemics of the disease. This hope was rudely shattered by the appearance of the disease in epidemic form in Tonkin and Hongkong, and a short time after in Kurrachee, Poonah and Bombay. In the last place alone 164,083 deaths occurred. Most important to us—and marking a new epoch in plague literature—was the first recorded appearance of the plague in the Western Hemisphere, in Santos, Brazil, in 1899. It even reached the port of New York, but was checked there by an efficient quarantine officer. The revival of the plague within the past eleven years has aroused universal interest. Since the outbreak at Hongkong, in 1894, the disease has appeared in many parts of the world. In India it has proved a terrible scourge since 1896. In the Punjab during the three years from 1901 to 1903, a million people died of it. For the year ending May, 1904, there were 913,784 deaths from this cause in India, an increase of more than 25,000 over 1903.

After an absence of more than two hundred years, plague obtained a foothold in Great Britain, and in Glasgow there was a small epidemic of short duration in the autumn of 1900. There have been a few cases at Mexican and South American ports. In San Francisco the plague smouldered for some time after March 6, 1900. During the twelve months ending June 30, 1904, there were twenty-four cases and twenty-three deaths; but after that time the disease disappeared from the city. As has been well illustrated in

Glasgow and San Francisco, the disease is readily held in check by proper sanitary measures.

Bubonic plague furnishes a striking illustration of the scientific advance of modern medicine. It was not until 1894 that positive knowledge of its true nature became known. Now its cause, method of propagation, and the means to prevent its spread are matters of scientific certainty. Dr. Kitasato discovered its cause in the form of a bacillus; it was found to be spread through the agency of insects and rodents, especially the rat; and Yersin and Haffkine discovered sera by which the cure and prevention of the disease could be accomplished. While during the great epidemic in India the mortality was from 90 to 95 per cent., it has been reduced in a subsequent epidemic by the use of Yersin's serum to 14 per cent. By the use of the Haffkine serum the number of people protected from acquiring the disease is from 95 to 100 per cent. (5).

Relief through modern science

That most hideous and terribly fatal disease, small-pox, had long been, previous to the eighteenth century, a terror and scourge to all classes throughout the world, and after the disappearance of the plague in England, became the severest epidemic disease of that country. A century ago one-tenth of all the people of the globe perished from small-pox, and nearly twice as many were permanently disfigured by its ravages. In England one person in every three was badly pock-marked, and 3,000 per each million of inhabitants died annually from the disease. In Bombay and Calcutta, from 1873 to 1876, 700,000 died from this disease (6). Shortly after the introduction of small-pox into Mexico by the Spaniards, it carried off over 3,500,000 of the natives. It is notable as illustrating the efficacy of intelligent health officers and an efficient quarantine service, that Australia and New Zealand have always remained exempt from this disease (6).

Losses due to small-pox

Perhaps the greatest of all sanitary triumphs occurring in the eighteenth century was Jenner's discovery of vaccination against small-pox. It was commenced in the year 1796, and although it was several years before it became general, its value as a preventive measure was not long in declaring itself by a steadily declining mortality. Thus, according

Relief through vaccination

to well authenticated returns, while the mortality in England was 88 per 1,000 deaths in the last ten years of the eighteenth century, it fell progressively from 64 to 11 per 1,000 deaths during the first six decades of the past century, as a result of the practice of vaccination (7). And if there are still recurrent outbreaks of the disease in England, it is because there are thousands of people living at the present day who have never been protected by vaccination, and many thousands more who have been imperfectly vaccinated. For it should be remembered that it was not until 1840 that England had any vaccination laws at all; not until 1853 that vaccination was provided gratuitously for the poor; and not until 1867 that vaccination was made compulsory amongst children generally. Occasional outbreaks may therefore be expected for years to come, especially in view of the increasing numbers of anti-vaccinationists; but that the disease can and will be finally eradicated is the belief as deep-rooted and strong in the minds of medical men and the educated public of the present day as it was in the heart of Edward Jenner.

In Prussia, compulsory vaccination has been enforced since April, 1875, with the result that small-pox has been practically **Effect of compulsory vaccination** annihilated, the mortality having been reduced to 0.36 per 100,000. In marked contrast to this are the French reports which show that from 1870 to 1895, over 20,000 have died from small-pox in Paris alone, where vaccination is not compulsory. A chart of the death rate in New York City is appended, showing the reduction since vaccination has been employed by the Department of Health (8). The recurrent waves reaching occasionally as high as 18 per 100,000 will undoubtedly return at intervals until compulsory and continuous vaccination is adopted.

The economic loss to a city from an epidemic of small-pox has been very well shown for Philadelphia by Dr. Lee, after the epidemic of 1871–72 (4). He considers the loss to travel and traffic on railroads, the loss to hotel-keepers, merchants and manufacturers from diminished patronage. He adds to these the cost of the care of the sick, the loss of time to them and to the state through their disability, and the expense of burial. Under these estimates the total cost of the epidemic was only a trifle less than twenty-two millions of dollars. Dr. Lee then gives a similar estimate of what might have been the expenditure under a policy of preventive measures. This would have necessitated the establishment of a vaccine bureau, with a large force of physicians for vaccinating

Economic saving through preventive measures

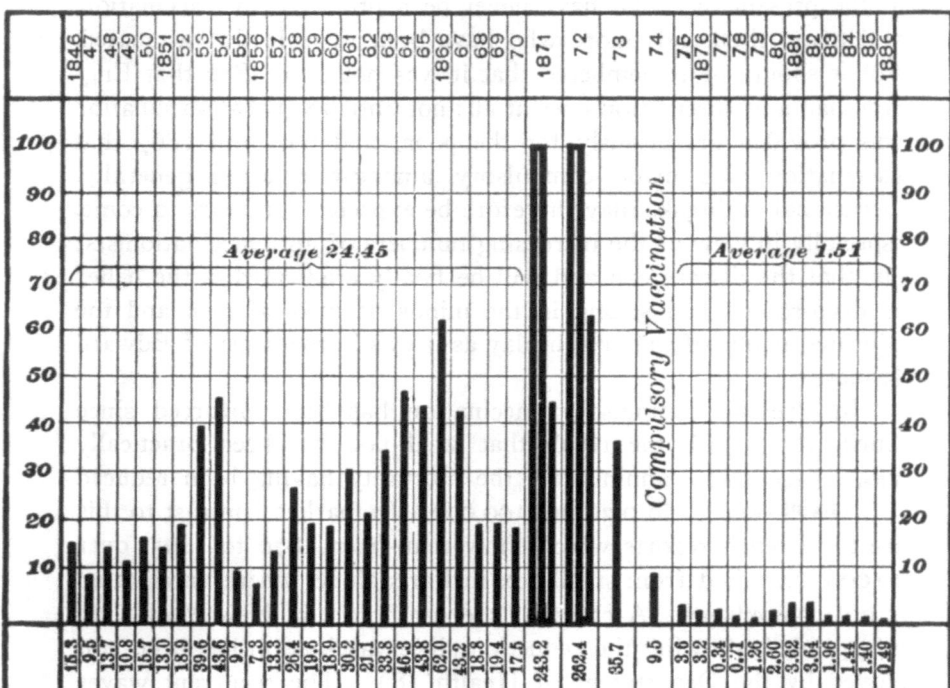

Progress of Small-Pox in Prussia Before and After the Enforcement of General Vaccination. Death-Rate Per 100,000 of Population. 1846–1886
Courtesy of W. B. Saunders & Co.

the public, a disinfecting station, with all its details, and the publication and distribution of pamphlets of instruction to the public. While the epidemic actually cost the city of Philadelphia about twenty-two million dollars, a policy of prevention, estimated in these details, would have cost about seven hundred thousand dollars. In other words, the sum total of this estimate leaves a balance to the credit of sanitation of over twenty-one million dollars.

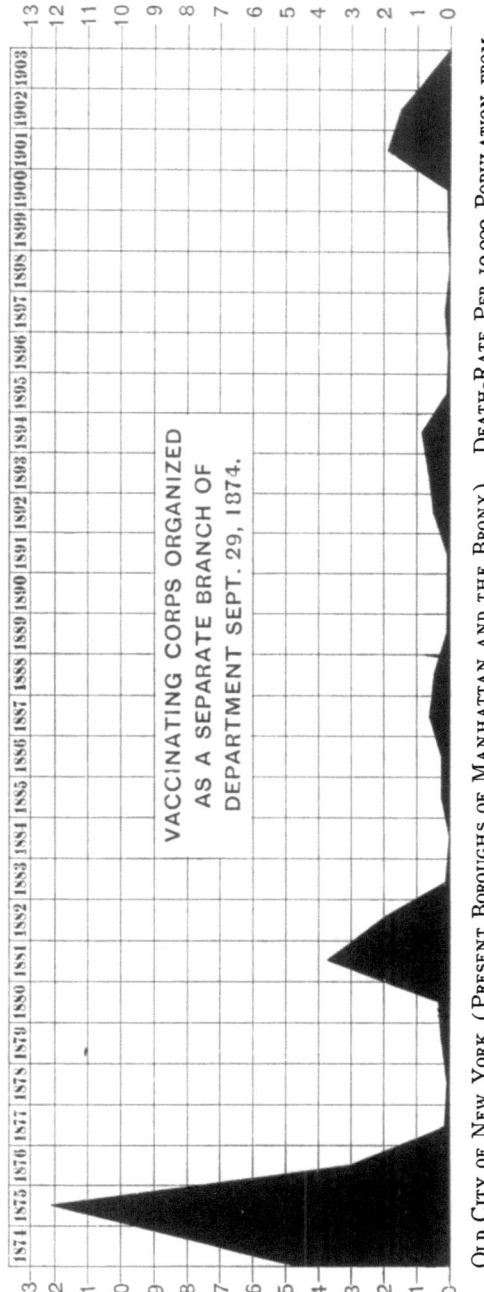

Old City of New York (Present Boroughs of Manhattan and the Bronx). Death-Rate Per 10,000 Population from Small-Pox. 1874–1903. Vaccinating Corps organized as a Separate Branch of Health Department, September 29, 1874

Courtesy of New York Board of Health

Few histories of epidemic diseases bring home more forcibly the devastation and loss from such causes, or illustrate the value **Losses due to yellow fever** of methods of prevention more clearly, than that of yellow fever. In 1800, in Spain, an epidemic of yellow fever was extremely desolating and mortal. Of the population of 57,499 in Cadiz, 48,520 were ill, and 7,387 died of the disease. Of 80,568 in Seville, 76,685 were attacked by the malady, and 14,685 died. Of 279,000 people in nine cities of the infected district in Spain, 77,500 died (9).

Between the years 1702 and 1878, yellow fever appeared in the United States, according to Keating, one hundred and twelve times, its invasions being most frequent and most destructive in the southern states, although they reached as far north as Nantucket Island, Mass. The first epidemic concerning which we have reliable information is that which visited Philadelphia in 1793. From the first of August to the middle of September of that year, 4,041 deaths occurred from this disease, in a city which originally contained but 40,144 inhabitants (10). During the next eighty years, the United States was visited by yellow fever every year but one. During this period two great epidemics occurred, one in New Orleans in 1853, and another in Norfolk in 1855. The most terrible visitation, however, was the epidemic of 1878 in Memphis and its vicinity. In this city of 19,500 people, there were 17,600 cases of yellow fever, with 6,000 deaths. An idea of the terrors of such an epidemic and its paralyzing effect on society and commerce may be drawn from the following description of this epidemic in Memphis by an eye witness (10):

By the last week in August the panic was over in the city. All had fled who could, and all were in camp who would go. There were then, it was estimated, about three thousand cases of fever—an appalling gloom hung over the doomed city. At night it was silent as the grave, by day it seemed desolate as the desert. There were hours, especially at night, when the solemn oppression of universal death bore upon the human mind, as if the day of judgment was about to dawn. Not a sound was to be heard; the silence was painfully profound. Death prevailed everywhere. Traffic and trade were suspended. The energies of all who remained were engaged in the struggle with death. The poor were reduced to beggary, and even the rich gladly accepted alms. . . . Even the animals felt the oppression and fled from the city. Rats, cats, or dogs were not to be seen. Death was everywhere triumphant. White women were seldom met with, children never. The voice of prayer was lifted up only at the bed of pain or death, or in some home circle where anguish was supreme and death threatened total annihilation. . . . Hundreds of men and women volunteered as nurses, who were destined to a speedy death. . . . A long line of graves in Elmwood Cemetery tells the story of their fidelity to a mission that was one purely of mercy and loving kindness.

The following will give an idea of the frightful mortality of this disease: During the epidemics since 1793, there have been 100,000 deaths from yellow fever. New Orleans has been the greatest sufferer with 41,348 deaths, followed by Philadelphia with 10,038, and Memphis with 7,759. New York has had 3,454 deaths. During our brief occupation of Cuba (July, 1898, to December, 1900) 1,575 cases of yellow fever ocurred, with 231 deaths. During the period from 1793 to 1900 there have been no less than 500,000 cases of yellow fever in the United States alone. Yet the actual loss of life from the disease, appalling as it is, is but a part of the distress which it has occasioned to the country. The pecuniary loss, both direct and indirect, is a matter of serious **Economic loss to the** moment. Keating states that the amount con-
country tributed by the world at large for the relief of the stricken cities of the South in 1878 was $4,548,703. Dr. Holbeck, chairman of the committee appointed in 1897 to investigate the cause of yellow fever, states in his report that the total loss to the country in the epidemic of 1878, was not less than $100,000,000. The loss to the city of New Orleans alone was over $10,000,000 (10).

In 1900, Major Walter Reed, working in Cuba on the United States Army Yellow Fever Commission, discovered that yellow **Relief through pre-** fever was transmitted by means of the mosquito,
ventive measures *Stegomyia fasciata,* and by this means only. Acting on this discovery, steps were taken to prevent further infection from this source by destruction of the insect, with the result that Cuba has since been free from this scourge, and it has been practically blotted out from our own southern states. General

Leonard Wood, at the memorial service in honor of **Major Reed**, who died soon after the completion of his work in Cuba, said: "I know of no man who has done so much for humanity, as Major Reed. His discovery results in the saving of more lives annually than were lost in the Cuban war, and saves the commercial interests of the world a greater financial loss in each year than the cost of the entire Cuban war."

Cholera probably originated in India many centuries ago. From India it first invaded Europe in 1826, and in 1831 spread to the Western Hemisphere and shortly extended over the greater part of the world. Several times since then the disease has spread to England, usually originating in India and Russia. The number of cases of illness and of deaths caused by these epidemics is appalling. During the epidemic of 1885 in Spain there were over one-third of a million cases with 120,000 deaths. In the year following, 100,000 deaths occurred from this disease in Japan. In the epidemic of 1892, 8,000 deaths occurred in the city of Hamburg. Upon that occasion the results of prevention by means of the filtration of a city's water supply were shown very strikingly; for while Altona and Hamburg, two adjoining cities, obtained their water supply from the same infected stream—the River Elbe—that used by Altona was filtered and that used by Hamburg was not. The enormous excess of the cases of sickness in Hamburg, over those in Altona, is shown in the accompanying chart (11), 17,000 cases occurring in Hamburg, while in Altona, although it got its water from the Elbe below Hamburg, after the river had received the sewage of 800,000 people, there were only 179 cases.

Losses due to cholera

Relief by preventive measures

In the year 1494, Charles VIII of France, in command of a large army, invaded Italy, and early in the following year besieged Naples. During the investment of the city syphilis broke out among the besiegers and spread rapidly throughout the army and later through the whole of Europe. At the present day syphilis is one of the most widely prevalent of all communicable diseases. The number of syphilitics in the United States has been estimated at 2,000,000 (6). The importance of the wide prevalence of this disease is due, not only to

Wide prevalence of syphilis

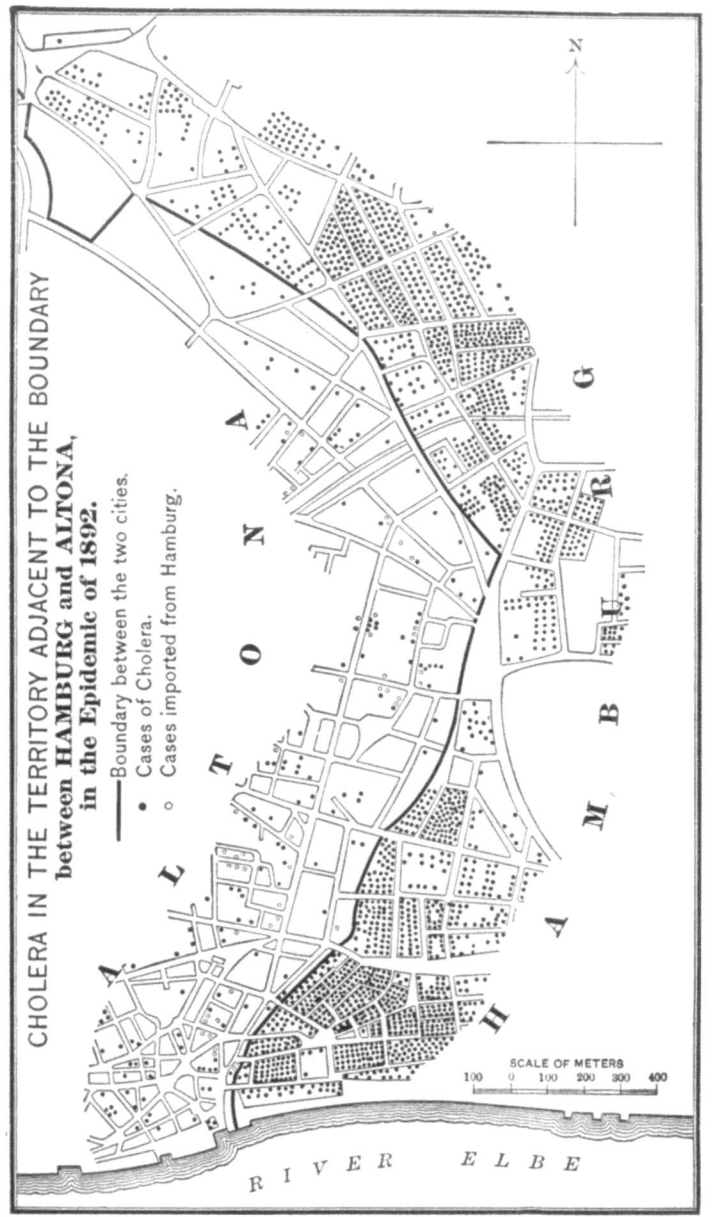

The two cities are practically one, the only sanitary difference in 1892 was that Hamburg used the unfiltered water from the Elbe and Altona filtered it

Courtesy of Rudolph Hering

the symptoms of the disease itself, but to the fact that it is the cause of a large number of diseases of the circulatory system and of diseases of the nervous system resulting in paralysis, imbecility or insanity.

The extent of venereal diseases in the English Army is enormous. In 100,000 men there were, in 1897, 10,631 cases of venereal disease. In 98,000 men in the British Navy, there were 11,193 cases. The loss to the English army in India from this cause is enormous, as shown by the following figures: In 60,000 men there were 16,789 cases in twelve months, with an average stay in the hospital of 30.79 days, representing a total loss of service of 514,-855 days. At Netley Hospital in England, in 1897, about one-third of all the patients were suffering from venereal diseases, the number of which showed an increase of 15 per cent. in fifteen years (12). Finally, the fatal results of syphilis are appreciated when we know that 15 per cent. of all deaths are due to diseases resulting from that condition, many of which affect the circulatory system (12). The cause and methods of transmission of these diseases are plainly known, and it should be one of the foremost tasks of preventive medicine to makes these diseases disappear from the world.

Far-reaching dangerous effects

Striking examples of types of disease which though not infectious are preventable, are scurvy and beri-beri; and the results which sanitary science has obtained in overcoming these scourges are among the most brilliant in the history of preventive medicine. Scurvy up to the latter half of the eighteenth century decimated the armies and fleets of Europe and often proved fatal among the civil population. It is a disease easily recognized and well defined; fostered, as many other diseases are, by insanitary conditions; but its real cause is insufficient food or a diet from which vegetables and fruit have been excluded, and therefore its prevention or cure depends upon a proper supply of vegetable food or vegetable juices. It is true all this had been known or surmised long anterior to the period in question; but it was reserved for Captain Cook, in his first voyage of discovery round the world, from 1772 to 1775, to prove beyond a doubt that the disease could be banished from every ship's crew,

Losses from scurvy

and that it could be entirely eradicated on land and sea. Hitherto it had been a cause of great mortality amongst seamen; and, to quote one instance out of many, in Anson's famous expedition some thirty years previous to that of Captain Cook, out of a total number of 900 hands, 600 died before the expedition returned, and chiefly from scurvy. During Captain Cook's three years' voyage, on the other hand, there were only four deaths, three from accident, and one from consumption, out of a total number of 118 men (7). Captain Cook thus earned for himself a foremost place among the sanitary reformers of the eighteenth century; but the nation took years to learn the lesson which he taught, and many more lives had to be sacrificed before it became compulsory that lime-juice should form a part of the commisariat of every sea-going vessel.

Relief through preventive measures

Beri-beri, an excruciatingly painful disease affecting the peripheral nerves, was for centuries the dread of Oriental armies and navies. In the troubles with Korea, in 1882, the efficiency of the Japanese navy was impaired almost 50 per cent. by this disease, and about one-third of the entire strength of the navy had been afflicted with the disease during the years from 1878 to 1883 inclusive. Following the cruise of the Japanese warship Kyujo, in 1883, during which 100 out of the 350 persons on board developed beri-beri, Takaki, who had discovered that the disease was due to an insufficiency of nitrogenous food, changed the dietary of the navy, with the result that from 1886 to 1893 not a single case developed, and during the war with Russia no case appeared in the floating force of over twenty-five thousand men. This triumph of Takaki's in overcoming beri-beri by preventive measures is one of the brilliant feats in modern medicine.

Losses from beri-beri

Relief through preventive measures

Of the infectious diseases capable of transmission, all are to a greater or less degree preventable. Even those diseases the causes of which are still unknown, *viz.*, yellow, typhus, and scarlet fever, trachoma, rabies, dengue, mumps, whooping-cough, measles, chicken-pox and small-pox, are capable to a large extent of being prevented. The list of preventable infectious diseases of known origin at the present time

Preventable infectious diseases

is a long one, and includes typhoid fever, cholera, tuberculosis, dysentery, pneumonia, diphtheria, meningitis, influenza, bubonic plague, syphilis, gonorrhœa, leprosy, tetanus, anthrax, actinomycosis, malaria, relapsing fever and diseases due to animal parasites. A brief *résumé* of a few of these diseases will show what progress has been made in reducing them in amount by various sanitary methods, what diseases still persist in large amount, and what diseases are increasing—thus accentuating the pressing need for further attempts at their prevention.

Typhoid fever is a disease which occurs as a result of the ignorance of the fact that the dejecta of typhoid fever patients contain **Losses from typhoid fever** the infective agent which may contaminate water and food, which when then swallowed by human beings may cause the disease anew. The amount of typhoid fever occurring in any locality is usually considered a good index of the knowledge and observance of sanitary principles, and the quality of the water supply. The reduction of this disease following the application of sanitary principles and the purification of the water supplies, illustrates more clearly than in any other case the direct results of methods of prevention; and the fact that many communities do not yet avail themselves of these methods gives an idea of the necessity for the education of the public and health-board and legislative officials, along these lines.

Typhoid epidemics have been extremely common during the last century and their frequency is apparently increasing in this country. Notable examples are those of Plymouth, Pa., in 1885, with 1,100 cases and 114 deaths, Ithaca, N. Y., in 1903, with 1,350 cases and 82 deaths, Watertown, N. Y., in 1904, with 582 cases and 44 deaths. During the past year there have been epidemics in Pittsburg, Pa., with 5,265 cases and 432 deaths, in Philadelphia, with 9,721 cases and 1,063 deaths, and in Scranton, Pa., with 1,155 cases and 111 deaths. These epidemics are allowed to occur in spite of the fact that it has been demonstrated that by attention to the drainage of soils and the introduction of pure water for domestic purposes, typhoid fever can be almost eliminated. No more striking instance of this can be cited than the remarkable reduction in the typhoid death-rate in the city of Munich. In 1856, the mortality from typhoid in Munich was 2.91 per 1,000 of population. At that time the soil of the city was honeycombed with cesspools, and a large part of the water supply was obtained from wells and pumps sunk in this soil. Between 1856 and 1887, the conditions of the city underwent, at several conspicuous periods, a radical sanitary reform. The cesspools were filled, and the introduction of new ones was prohibited. An elaborate system of sewers was introduced, pumps and wells were abandoned, and a pure water supply was brought from a source beyond suspicion of pollution. As a result the mortality from typhoid fever fell, and in 1887 it had reached the very low rate of 0.1 per 1,000 of population, a reduction of about 96.6 per cent. in the deaths from this disease alone (11).

Relief through preventive measures

The reduction in the mortality from typhoid fever as a result of filtration of the city water supply is strikingly shown in the accompanying illustrations, in the case of Berlin, Magdeburg, and Breslau. Another table shows the amount of typhoid fever resulting from several different kinds of water supply, and another the amount of typhoid fever still prevalent in New York City—an amount capable of far greater reduction.

In the Boer war the British army in South Africa lost 7,991 men from typhoid fever, the number of men dying from wounds received in battle being only 7,852. In the Spanish-American war the report of the Commission shows that one-fifth of the soldiers in our national encampments had typhoid fever,—among 107,973 men there were 20,738 cases with 1,580 deaths. So slight has been the improvement in the principles of sanitary administration in the army, due to lack of proper system and education and suitably trained men, that should we engage in another war to-morrow this horrible record would, without a shadow of a doubt, be repeated.

Typhoid in our armies

Recurrence threatened

In striking contrast to this is the result in the Japanese army during the recent war with Russia, in which the greatest enlightenment prevailed on the part of the Japanese in regard to methods for the prevention of disease.

Lesson from the Japanese

22   Education and Preventive Medicine

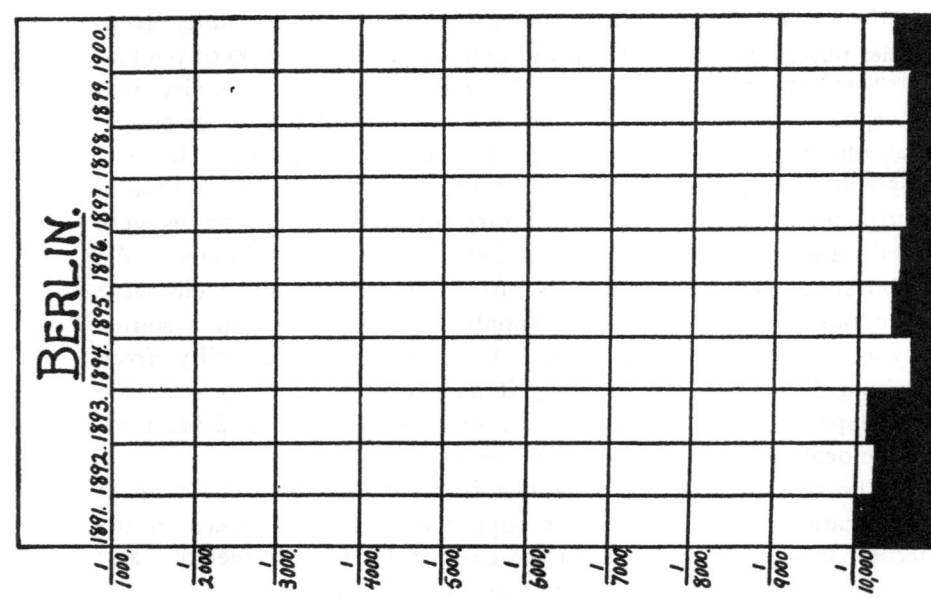

Filtered Municipal Water Supply

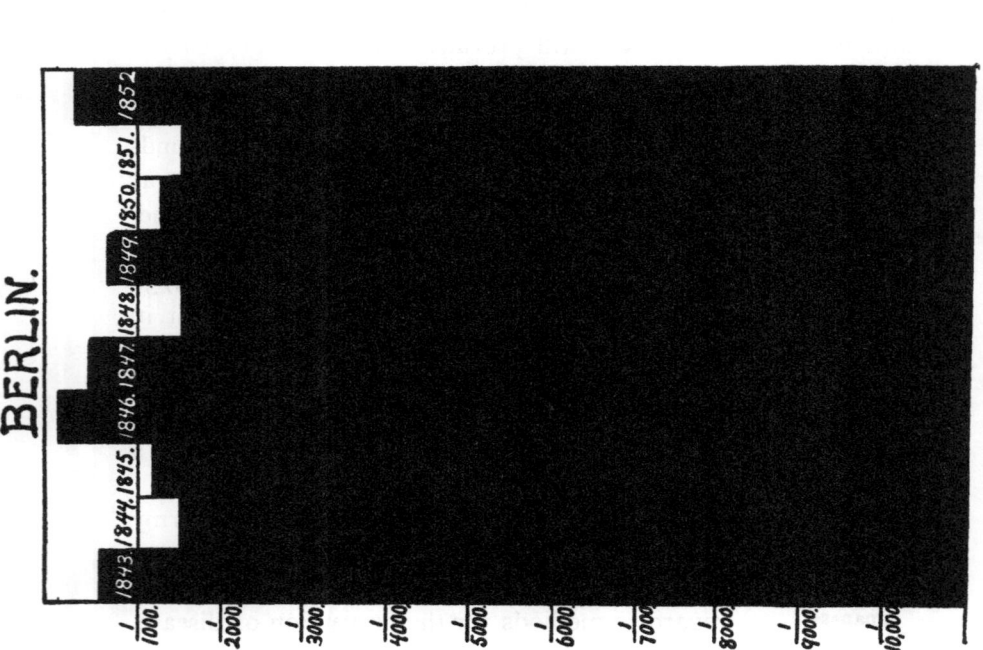

Unfiltered Municipal Water Supply

New York Medical Journal, Nov. 29, 1902. Courtesy of Dr. A. Seibert

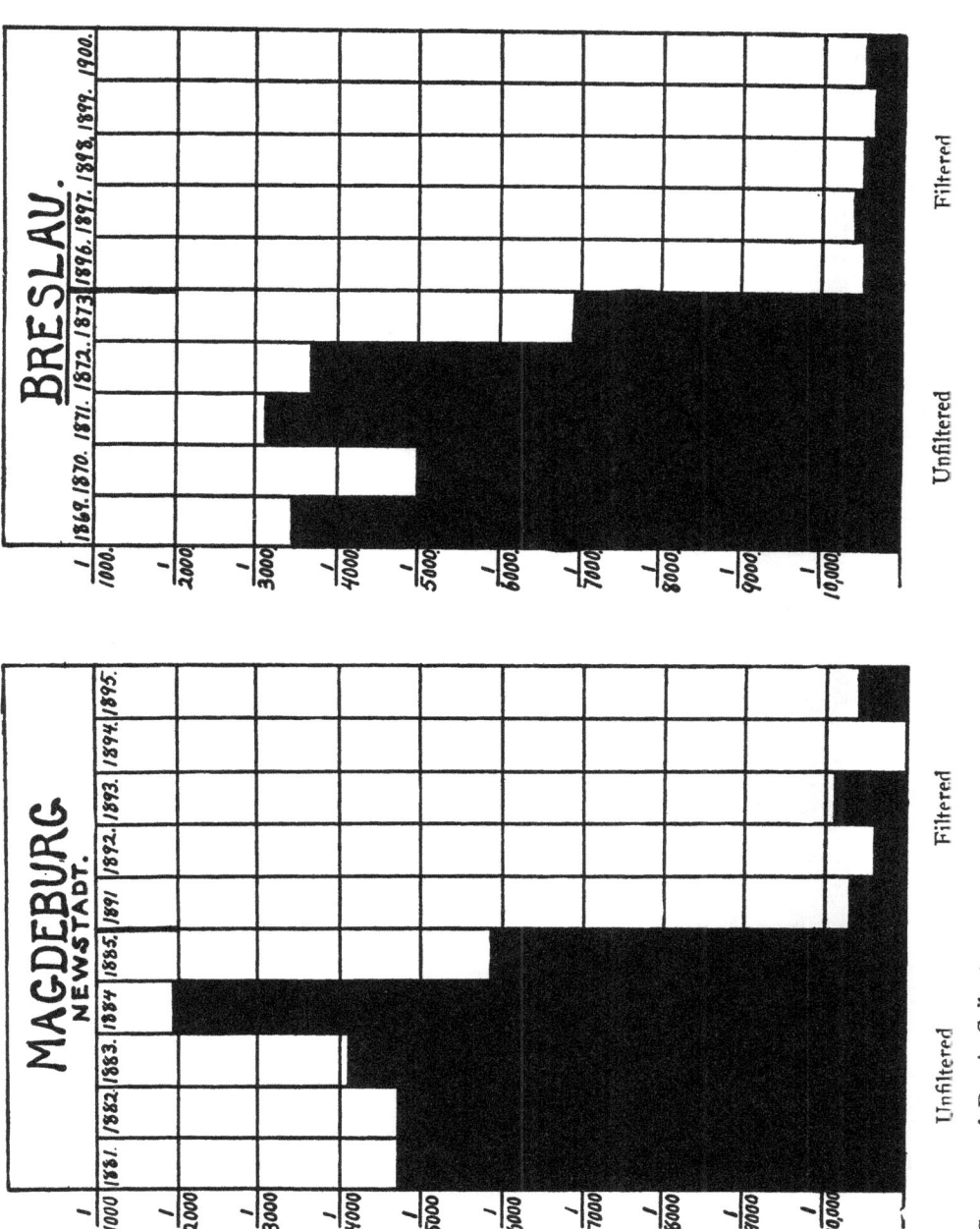

Courtesy of Dr. A. Seibert

24   *Education and Preventive Medicine*

The total of typhoid fever cases was only 187 in General Oku's army of 100,000 men during a seven months active campaign. A notable result which the Japanese obtained by their knowledge and application of measures of prevention, was the reduction of dysentery from 12,052 cases in the war with China, to 6,624 in the

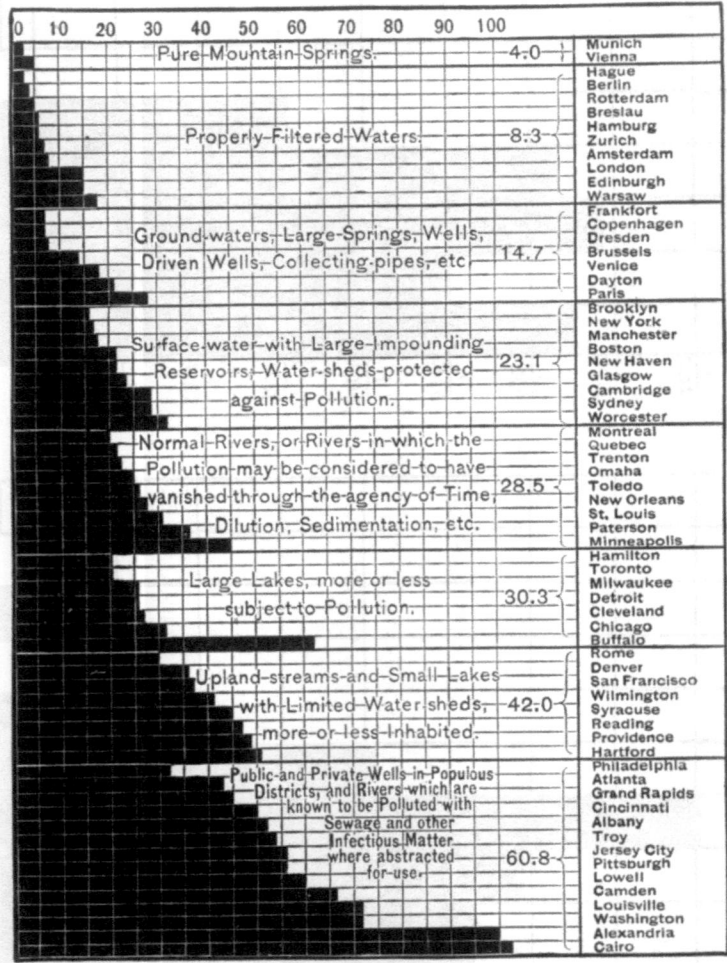

DEATH-RATES FROM TYPHOID FEVER IN 1894 IN 50 CITIES. Grouped According to Quality of Drinking Water

Courtesy of Lea & Febiger

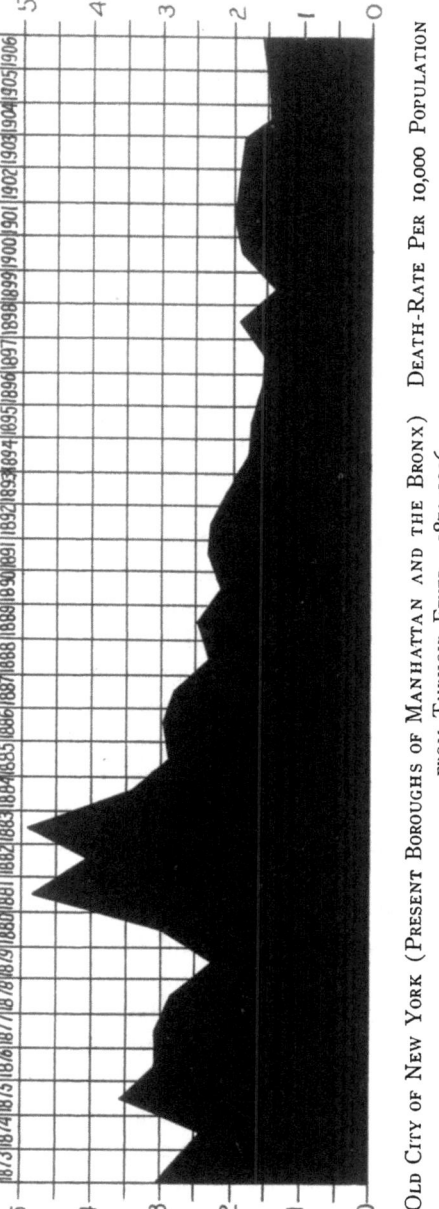

Old City of New York (Present Boroughs of Manhattan and the Bronx) Death-Rate Per 10,000 Population from Typhoid Fever. 1873–1906

Courtesy of New York Board of Health

Russian war, of cholera from 7,667 cases to none, and of malaria from 41,734 to 1,257; and this great reduction was obtained notwithstanding the fact that the army in the Russian war was three times the size of that in the Chinese war (13).

The cost of typhoid fever each year in sickness and death throughout America amounts to many millions of dollars. The sickness and death from this cause in New York City and in the epidemics in Philadelphia, Scranton, Pittsburg, during the past year represent an economic loss to those cities of $3,750,000, counting the value of each life lost at $1,500, the duration of the sickness, twenty-eight days, and the average daily wage, $1.50, and excluding the cost of nursing, medicines, etc. Such epidemics, with their resulting losses, occurring under our very eyes, are startling in an age which is considered enlightened. Proper instruction of the public and of health and legislative authorities, with the application of well-known methods of prevention, would result in a very great saving from loss by this disease and banish it forever into the background.

Economic loss from recent epidemics

Within the past few years the public has begun to awaken to a realization of the vast destruction of human life caused by tuberculosis. Popular agitation has done much to show what can be accomplished by methods of organization and education, but has emphasized still more strongly the need for further measures along this line. The greatest activity in preventing this disease is justified when the extent of the damage done by it is known, as illustrated by the following facts:

Losses due to tuberculosis

More than one-third of all the deaths that occur between the ages of 15 and 35 are due to the Great White Plague (2). It is a waste of youth prepared for life and labor, cut off by needless death as life and labor begin. A prominent physician said a few years ago: "This is a disease which has claimed more victims than all the wars and all the plagues and scourges of the human race. The annual tribute of the United States to this scourge is over one hundred thousand of its inhabitants. Each year the world yields up one million ninety-five thousand, each day three thousand, each minute two, of its people, as a sacrifice to this plague. Of the seventy-two million individuals now peopling these

United States, ten millions must inevitably die of this disease if the present ratio is kept up."

The economic loss is no less striking than the above figures, and illustrates the immense saving almost within our grasp, which will accrue from well-directed measures of prevention. Considering that 10,000 people every year die of tuberculosis in New York City, the annual loss to the city is $15,000,000. The cost of their nursing, food, medicines, attendance, as well as the loss of productive labor, adds a further loss to the municipality of $8,000,000. Upon the same basis it is estimated that the annual loss in the United States from tuberculosis alone is $330,000,000 a year. Illinois has figured its loss from this disease at $36,551,800, Iowa at $14,620,000, and Maryland at $10,000,000 a year (14).

Economic loss from tuberculosis

The mortality from tuberculosis is, therefore, a problem compared with which all other social problems of a medical character sink into insignificance. The prevention of a large portion of the mortality from the disease is within our power, and is justly deserving of the solicitude, the active personal interest, and the liberal pecuniary support of all who have the real welfare of the people at heart. Our efforts in this direction are stimulated by the success which has already been attained, as illustrated by the accompanying charts. Since 1886, the death-rate for Greater New York has decreased 40 per cent. This means an annual saving of 6,000 lives; but the loss to the city from tuberculous diseases is still enormous. Relief can be accomplished through measures of hygiene, popular education, isolation, laws, and the application of discoveries by laboratory research.

Relief by preventive measures

The diminution in the occurrence of diphtheria illustrates very well the influence of modern scientific developments resulting from laboratory research combined with intelligent hygienic measures. This has been brought about by the use of diphtheria antitoxin. Previous to the antitoxin period, the mortality ranged from 40 to 50 per cent.; since its introduction it has fallen to less than 10 per cent. (15). The diminution in the mortality of

Diphtheria

Antitoxin and hygiene

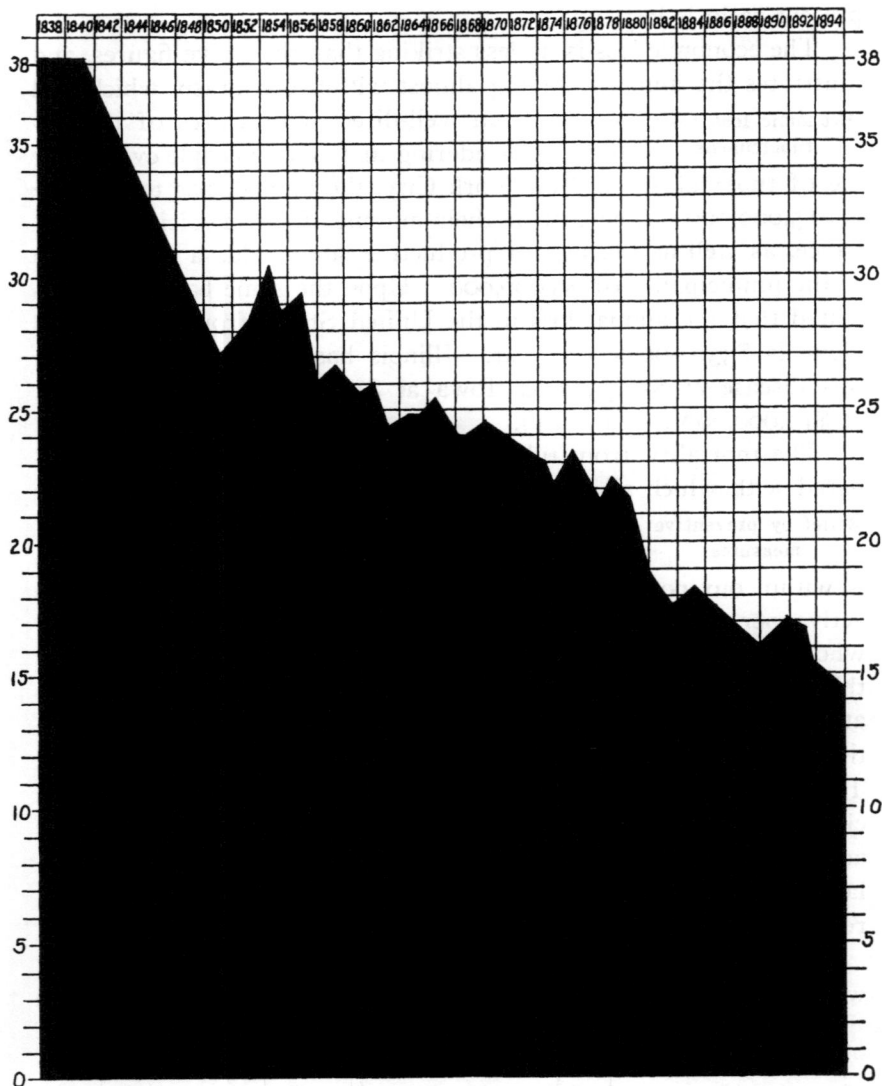

Death-Rate from Phthisis in England and Wales Per 10,000 Living
1838–1894

Courtesy of Swan, Sonnenschein & Co.

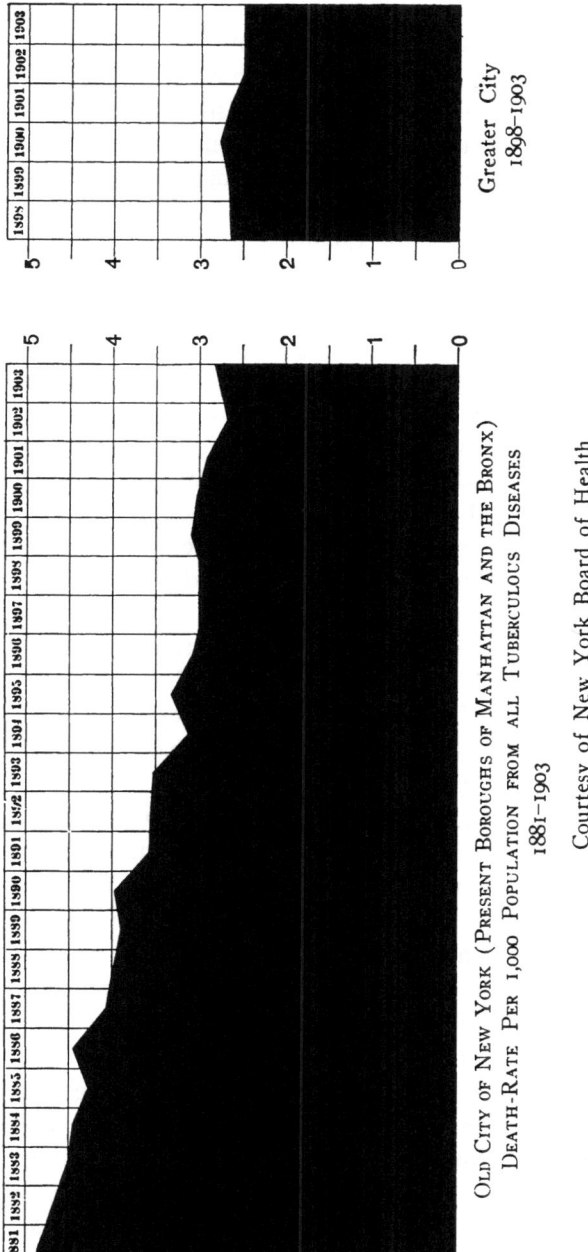

Old City of New York (Present Boroughs of Manhattan and the Bronx)
Death-Rate Per 1,000 Population from all Tuberculous Diseases
1881–1903

Greater City 1898–1903

Courtesy of New York Board of Health

diphtheria has been nothing short of marvelous; but armed with the weapons we now possess, no child should die of diphtheria. The accompanying chart illustrates how the death-rate from this disease in New York has been diminished during the last decade. The fact that the mortality is still 60 per 100,000, shows the necessity for more general application of our knowledge of the prevention of this disease.

The effect of modern scientific principles and efficient public sanitary control in curbing a noxious disease is perhaps nowhere better illustrated than in the case of rabies. **Losses due to rabies** Rabies, or hydrophobia, is a very widespread disease, and during the last century has inflicted severe losses throughout Europe and in America. At the present time it is known in almost every country on the globe, Australia being the only one which is absolutely exempt, owing to the rigid quarantine enforced against the importation of dogs. It is most common in Belgium, Russia and France, 7,083 cases having occurred from 1895 to 1898, inclusive, in the last named country. In England it has from time to time been widespread, but at present, owing to strict measures, it has been practically stamped out. The money losses from the occurrence of rabies in live stock in this country are very great. When untreated it is a very fatal disease, according to Tordieu, Thamhayn and Bonley, 46.6 per cent. of the cases ending fatally. Since the commencement of the Pasteur preventive treatment some 55,000 persons have been inoculated. The total average mortality is 0.77 per cent. During the year 1899 the mortality of cases treated at the Institute in Paris was 0.25 per cent.

As regards both man and animals the most rational procedure for prevention is to attempt the eradication of the disease; and since **Relief by preventive measures** it is kept alive by the canine races our measures must be directed to the control of dogs. The results obtained by strict enforcement of muzzling seem to justify its recommendation. To this measure is ascribed the eradication of the disease from Berlin in the year 1854–1855, and the recent results obtained in Great Britain are most striking. The accompanying table illustrates the diminution of the disease following

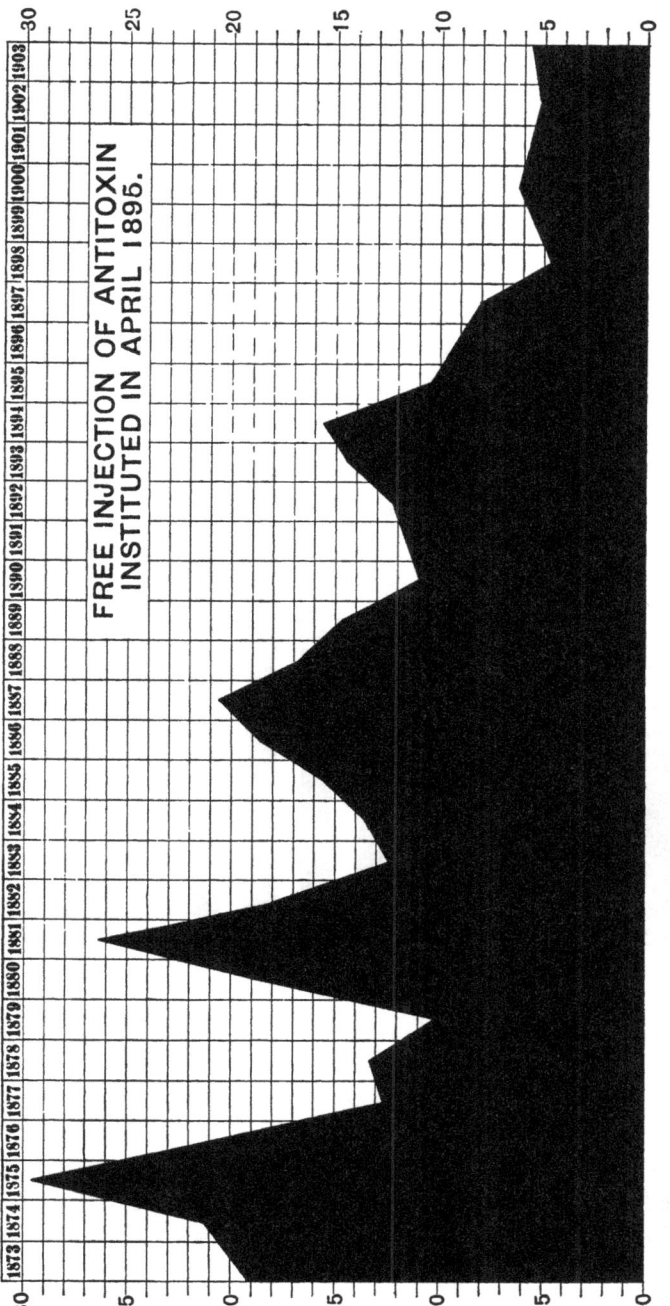

Old City of New York (Present Boroughs of Manhattan and the Bronx). Death-Rate Per 10,000 Population from Diphtheria and Croup. 1873–1903. Free injection of Antitoxin Instituted in April, 1895

Courtesy of New York Board of Health

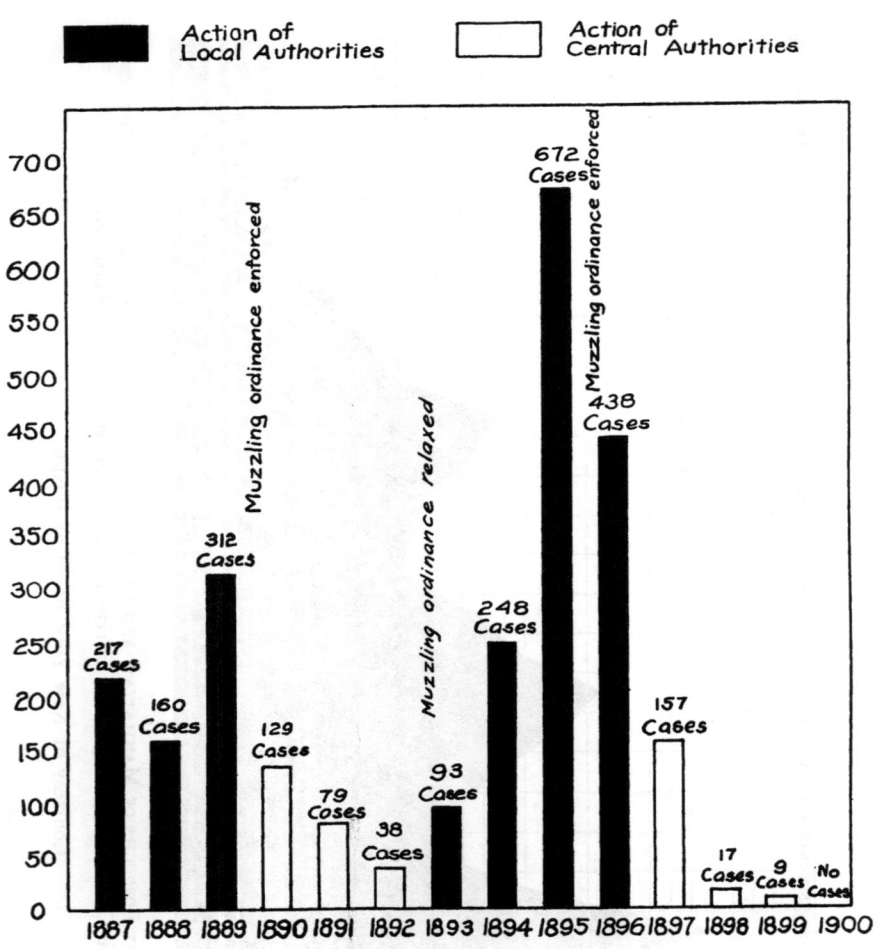

PREVENTION OF RABIES

TABLE SHOWING EFFECT OF ENFORCEMENT OF MUZZLING BY CENTRAL AUTHORITIES IN ENGLAND. 1887–1900

Courtesy of Mazyck P. Ravenel, M.D.

muzzling, as well as the increase whenever the muzzling ordinances were relaxed (16). The fact that during the past year the occurrence of rabies has reached enormous proportions in Massachusetts, due to some extent to lack of administrative control and popular ignorance, accentuates very strongly the necessity for the adoption of measures which will lead to the prevention of this disease.

Malaria, though a disease which usually responds easily to medical treatment, has been one of the serious menaces to commerce and society on account of its widespread prevalence. In the past, entire districts have been made uninhabitable by its presence. An army surgeon, Major Ross, acting upon the suggestion of Sir Patrick Manson, demonstrated the fact that the malarial organism is transported by a genus of mosquito, *Anopheles,* and transmitted by the bite of infected mosquitoes of this group. Acting upon this knowledge it has since been possible, by destroying these insects and their breeding places, to reclaim vast areas for the uses of civilization and to diminish effectually the prevalence of this disease. The problems involved in this process are those which occur within the realms of civil and sanitary engineering, and require special training of a kind best acquired in a school of public health and preventive medicine.

Malaria and prevention

The prevalence and mortality of the contagious diseases, scarlet fever and measles, etc., in America and Europe, constitute them the great dreaded scourges of childhood. It is estimated from the records of the London Fever Hospital that about six hundred thousand cases of these diseases, which are perfectly well understood to be preventable, occur in that country every year (4). The following charts show the prevalence of scarlet fever and measles in New York, the reduction in the amount since the institution of quarantine, and the amount which still persists.

Prevalence of exanthemata

Prevention by quarantine

Gonorrhœa is a very widespread disease, though preventable, and is concerned most intimately with questions of public morality and its control. A part of this question which is not frequently considered, however, is its effect on public and private charities, in its connection with the maintenance of institutions for the blind. It is reckoned that of the total blindness affecting people, about one-half is due to inflammation of the eyelids (purulent conjunctivitis), a very large proportion of which cases are gonorrhœal in origin (17). A large num-

Gonorrhœa and preventable blindness

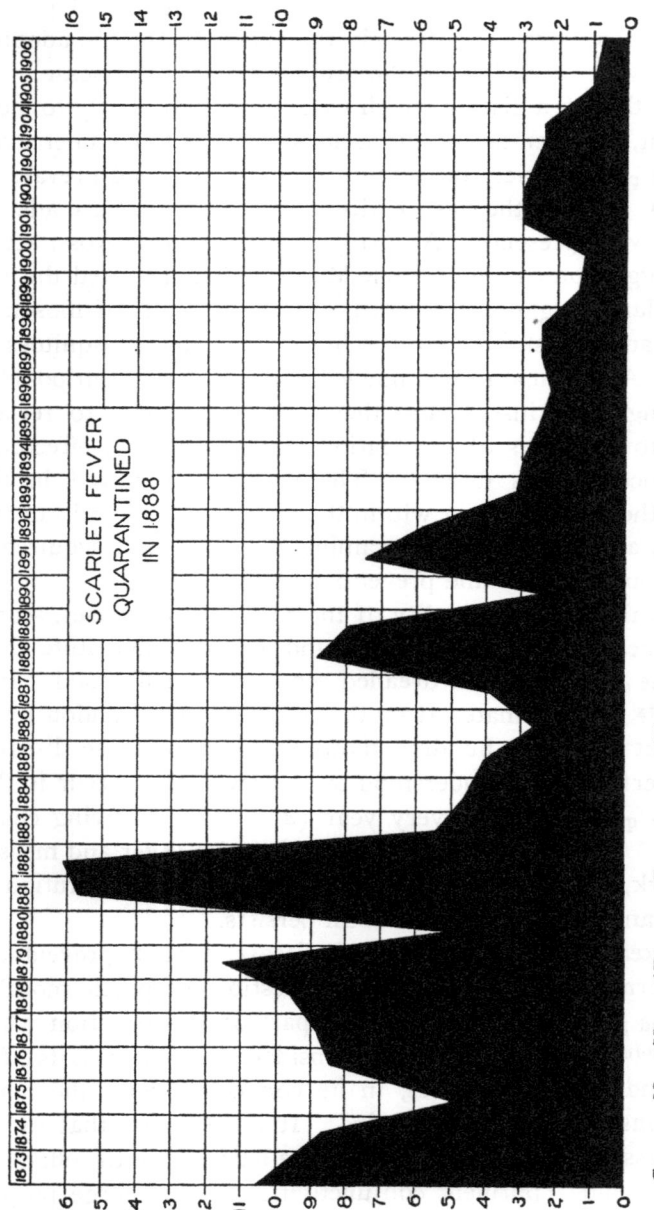

Old City of New York (Present Boroughs of Manhattan and the Bronx). Death-Rate Per 10,000 Population from Scarlet Fever. 1873–1906. Scarlet Fever Quarantined in 1888

Courtesy of New York Board of Health

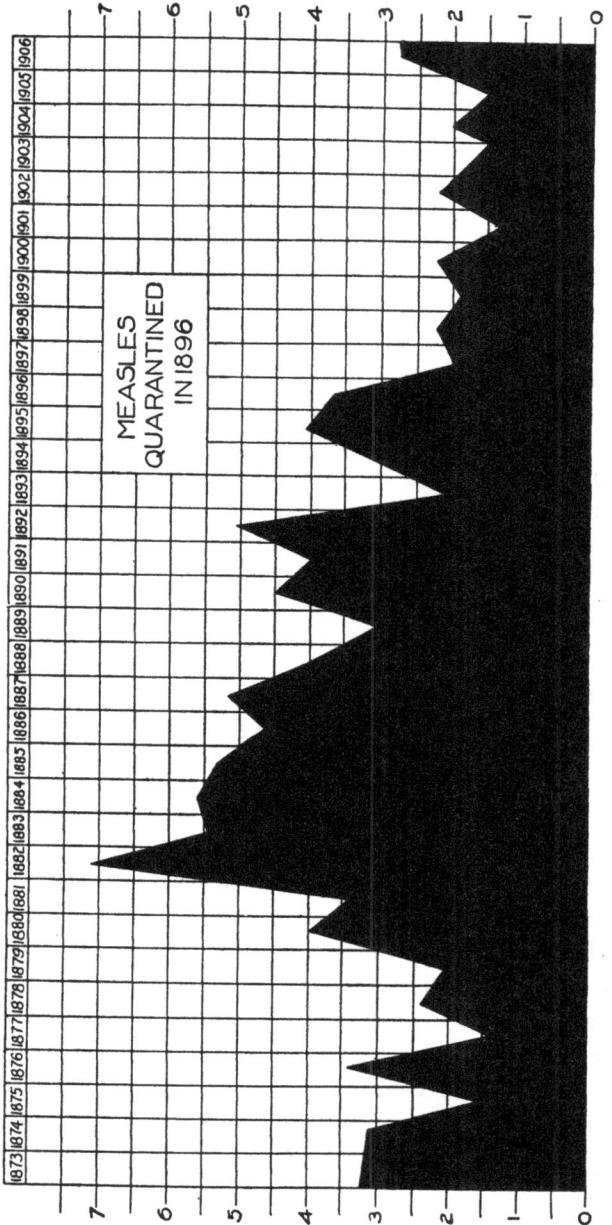

Old City of New York (Present Boroughs of Manhattan and the Bronx). Death-Rate Per 10,000 Population from Measles. 1873–1906. Measles Quarantined in 1896

Courtesy of New York Board of Health

ber of these cases occur at the time of birth, and means of prevention are simple and easy if known. Proper education in this one fact alone would save a large part of the cost of our institutions for the blind and save for active careers those condemned to lifelong darkness.—Of all conditions of pelvic inflammation in women, it has been estimated that 75 per cent. are due to gonorrhœal infection and are preventable.

In North America it is estimated that from one-fourth to one-third of all the deaths in a community are those of children under **Preventable death in New York children** one year of age; and in New York alone, during the summer months, 50 per cent. of the deaths occur among babies of this age (4). By far the larger proportion of these deaths are preventable and are directly traceable to improper conditions of food and drink, which a better understanding of hygiene would correct. The death-rate in some tenement house districts in New York runs as high as 204 per 1,000. Four or five times as many babies die in these houses as in the houses of the well-to-do districts.

A great deal is being done to reduce this fearful mortality, and the deepest impress which has been made upon the average death-rate of cities has been in the reduction of infant mortality through a better understanding of its causes, with especial reference to a clean milk supply. By such means as have been at our disposal there has been brought about a decrease in deaths of children under one year of age from 240 per thousand in 1891 to 145 per thousand in 1903, and in children under five years of age, from 96 per thousand in 1891 to 55 per thousand in 1903—an immense reduction. **Marked reduction of death-rate through preventive measures** There are few other fields of preventive medicine where the factor of education of the public and of those officials occupying positions on health-boards and sanitary and milk commissions is such an important one as here.

When, in any civilized community, the loss from any disease is increasing, that fact becomes of immense concern to the community, especially when the disease falls within the category of preventable diseases. **Increase of pneumonia** For the past thirty years, there has been a constant increase in New York in the death-rate from pneumonia. This became a matter of so much concern that in 1904 a commission was appointed by the Mayor of New York to investigate the subject of respiratory diseases, in the hope that added information could be obtained which

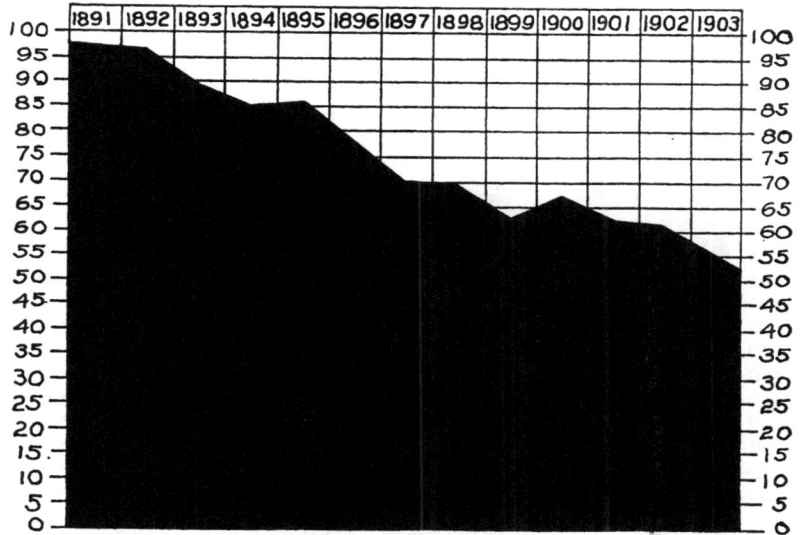

OLD CITY OF NEW YORK—DEATH-RATE OF CHILDREN UNDER FIVE YEARS PER 1,000 OF ESTIMATED POPULATION AT THAT AGE. 1891–1903
Courtesy of New York Board of Health

would lead to the staying of this increasing mortality. The cause of pneumonia is known, as well as much in regard to the method of transmission. It is a widespread disease, sparing no class or condition, and has been in recent years the cause of the loss to the country of many of its most brilliant workers.

During 1900, there were 105,971 deaths in the United States from this disease; that is, of every 1,000 deaths, 106 were due to **Great losses from** pneumonia. This ratio had increased since **pneumonia** 1890 from 90.6 per 1,000 (14). While the death-rate from tuberculosis has decreased since 1860, 39.5 per cent., the death-rate from pneumonia has *increased* 349 per cent. There is some decrease in the death-rate in the country districts, but an overwhelming increase in the centers of population (14). Pneumonia is essentially, then, a disease of our modern conditions of crowding, and must be met by modern weapons of defence.

Its relation to other diseases is clearly shown in the reports from Iowa and Illinois. Iowa is essentially a country community,

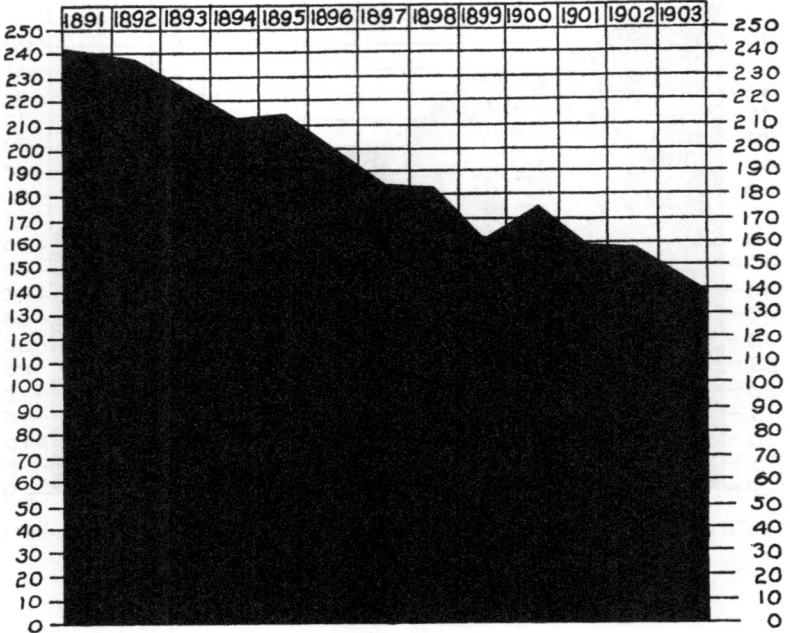

OLD CITY OF NEW YORK (PRESENT BOROUGHS OF MANHATTAN AND THE BRONX) DEATH-RATE OF CHILDREN UNDER ONE YEAR PER 1,000 OF ESTIMATED POPULATION AT THAT AGE. 1891–1903

Courtesy of New York Board of Health

having but one city of over 40,000 population, yet pneumonia carries off yearly more children than any other one disease, nearly eight times as many as consumption. Chicago, with a population somewhat approximating that of Iowa, in 1900 had 3,611 deaths from pneumonia—one-eighth of all its fatalities. This was twice the rate for rural Iowa. Illinois has double the population of Iowa and four times the number of deaths from pneumonia. In Chicago, pneumonia claimed 33 per cent. more than tuberculosis, 44 per cent. more than all other contagious diseases combined (14). There are more deaths from this disease under the age of five years than from any other disease—nearly twelve thousand more than cholera infantum. Not so much a question of race suicide as a question of child murder—a slaughter of the innocents!

To conquer this disease all modern resources must be brought **Pneumonia a preventable disease** into play. Not only are questions of public sanitation and education involved, but an immense amount of research in questions concerning the production **Need for further research** of immunity. The procedure not only holds out great promise for the alleviation of the condition, but gives encouragement of relief in the not far distant future.

Cerebrospinal meningitis is another disease which most urgently commands our attention; not only because it has of recent years **Increase of meningitis** been increasing by bounds, but because it is the cause of the most excrutiating suffering that man has ever fallen heir to, and, while generally fatal, those cases which survive are spared, as a rule, only to live a life of imbecility or feeble-mindedness. The cause of the disease is known. It seems to have a predilection for those with depressing mental and bodily surroundings, and is especially liable to occur among the misery and squalor of the large tenement houses in cities. Hence it, too, like pneumonia, resolves itself into one of our typical modern medical problems. The accompanying chart illustrates its enormous increase in New York in the year 1905. The cause being known, cerebrospinal meningitis is a preventable disease, but in order to overcome it the same help must be solicited from all known and modern methods of prevention, as in the case of pneumonia.

The preceding *résumé* has been devoted to a large extent to the preventable infectious diseases. There are other diseases, however, demanding attention, which though arising from causes imperfectly or not at all known, challenge our best efforts at prevention. This is the case especially with such of those diseases as are on the increase, and it is particularly true, for this reason, of cancer, diabetes, heart disease, and Bright's disease.

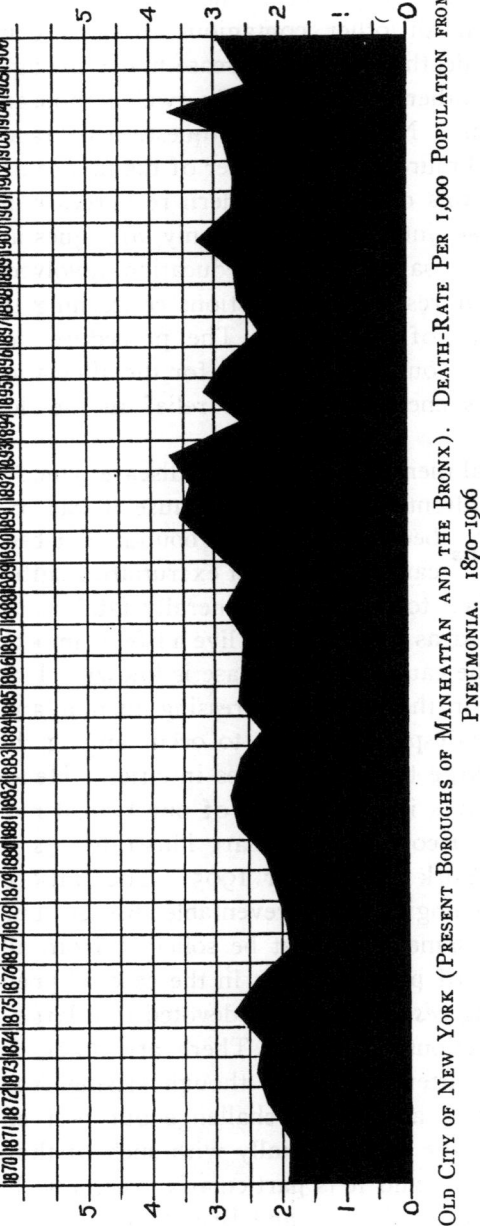

Old City of New York (Present Boroughs of Manhattan and the Bronx). Death-Rate Per 1,000 Population from Pneumonia. 1870–1906

Courtesy of New York Board of Health

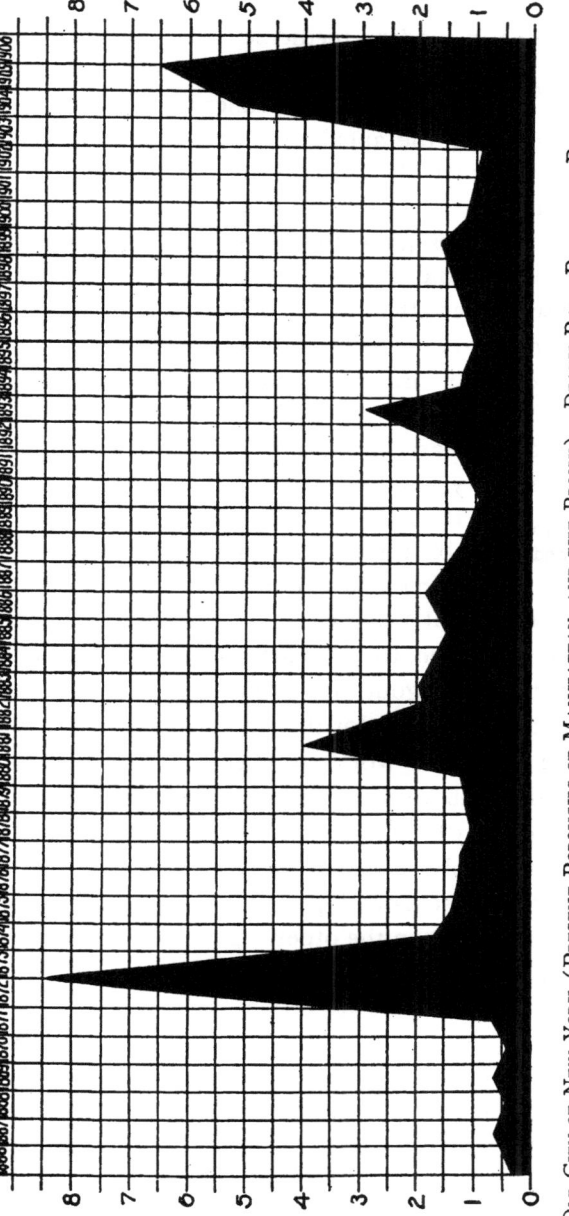

Old City of New York (Present Boroughs of Manhattan and the Bronx). Death-Rate Per 10,000 Population from Cerebrospinal Meningitis. 1866–1906

Courtesy of New York Board of Health

The prevalence of cancer at the present day is one of the most startling conditions in modern medicine. Reference to the accompanying chart, showing Newsholme's estimate of the increase of cancer in England since 1860 (18), prepares one for the appalling fact that at the present day, of all persons who reach the age of thirty-five years, one in every 21 men, and one in every 12 women, eventually die of cancer. Modern activity has been great in research for the cause of cancer, at present unknown, and the seriousness of the subject justifies further efforts wherever attempts are being made to prevent disease. Charity can seldom act to better advantage than by lessening or obviating the years of suffering and misery preceding death by cancer.

Prevalence of cancer

Diabetes, heart disease and Bright's disease have been rapidly increasing in recent years, probably as a result of our modern method of living. In each case the rate has doubled within the past thirty years—the accompanying chart illustrating this in the case of heart disease and Bright's disease. These latter frequently occur as a secondary condition to processes of known cause, and like chronic rheumatism and gout, are often concerned with some perversion of nutrition. Hence, for their final solution and prevention, we are thrown upon the work of chemical investigation, which must be pursued in laboratories having close connection with hospitals where diseases of the type under consideration are received. This illustrates as keenly as any other type of disease the important connection between a school of preventive medicine on one hand, and hospital laboratories on the other. The latter must be supplied, if many of our present obscure problems of prevention are to be solved.

Increase of diabetes, heart disease and Bright's disease

In recent years it has been brought to the attention of the medical profession and those interested in charitable reforms that a great deal of the disease and incompetency of adult life could be prevented by eradicating the underlying causes in childhood. Access to children for this purpose is most readily attained in the public schools and for this reason

Physical defect starting in childhood

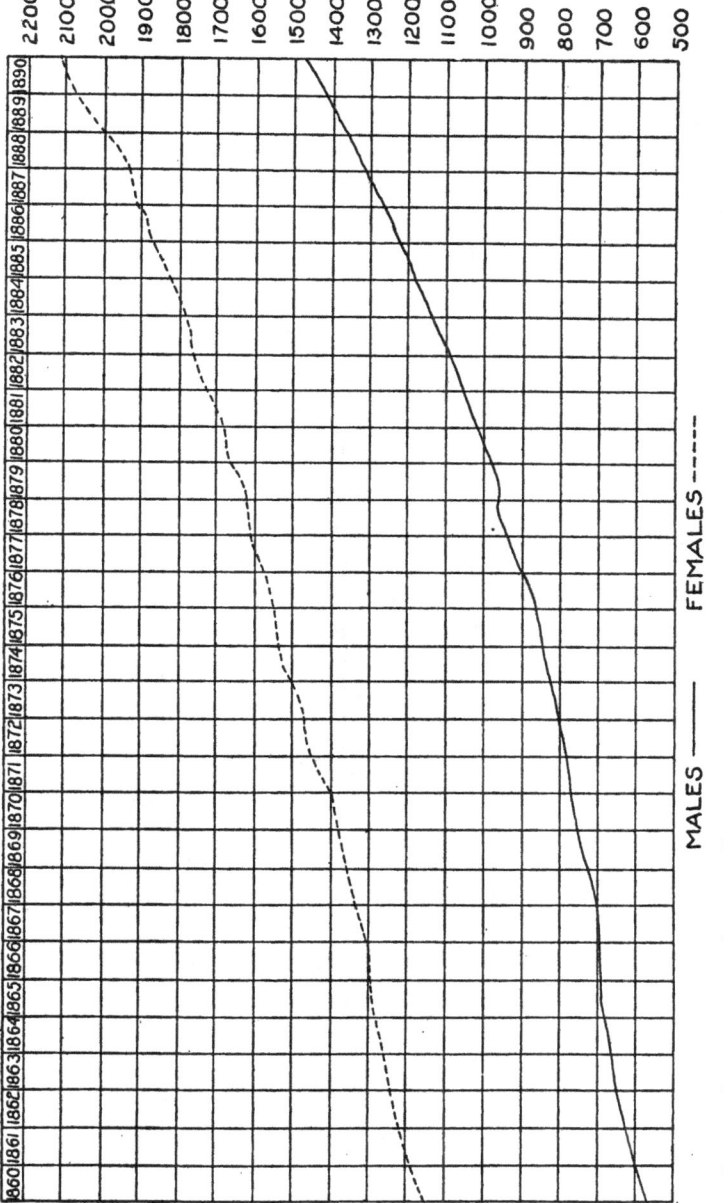

Curves Showing the Annual Deaths from Cancer Per Million Living, Aged 25 and Upwards, in England 1860–1890

From Newsholme's Vital Statistics

44   *Education and Preventive Medicine*

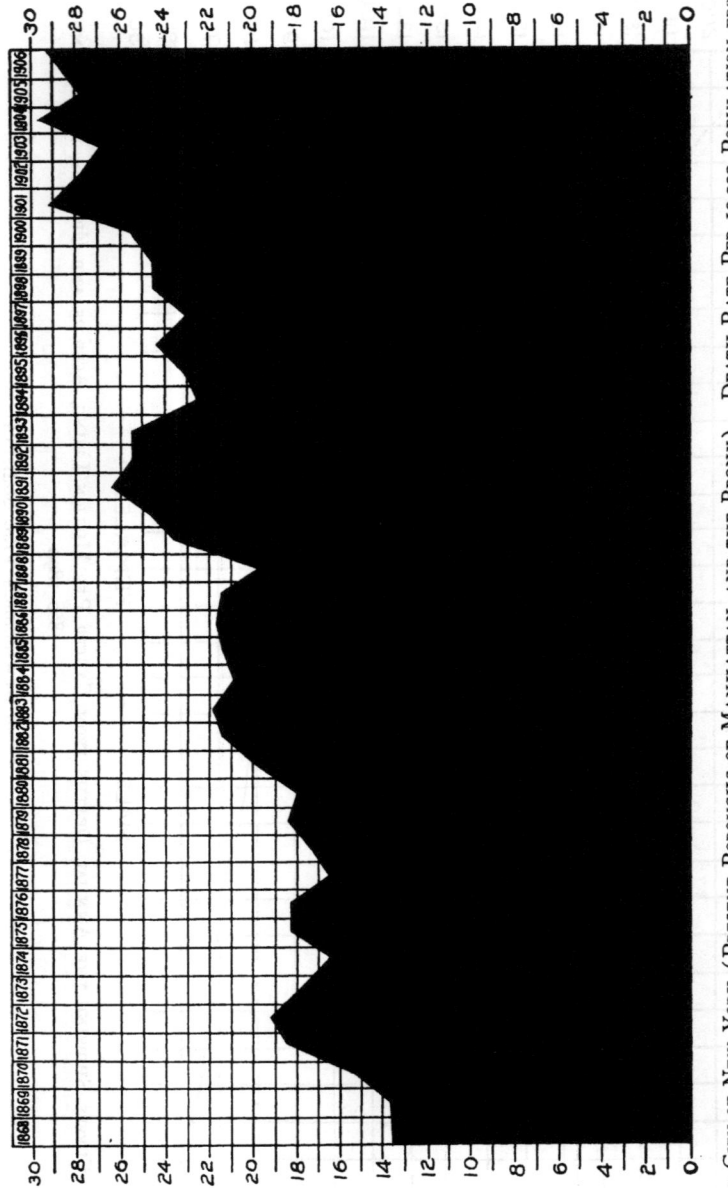

Old City of New York (Present Boroughs of Manhattan and the Bronx). Death-Rate Per 10,000 Population from Bright's and Heart Diseases Combined. 1868–1906

Courtesy of New York Board of Health

the movement has recently culminated in the formation of a Committee on the Physical Welfare of School Children. This committee found that of

One hundred thousand New York school children examined

66 per cent. needed medical or surgical attention or better nourishment

40 per cent. needed dental care

38 per cent. had enlarged cervical glands

31 per cent. had defective vision

18 per cent. had enlarged tonsils

10 per cent. had post-nasal growths

6 per cent. were undernourished

These conditions of physical defect are not only causes of future disease, but are found to interfere with the child's best mental development and capability of rapid assimilation of educational training. Efforts have been made to remedy these defects where found, with the most gratifying results in the way of increased efficiency in the children's application to work and steadier attendance. Corrective measures are provided largely through the means of the public boards of health, but the necessity still exists of training public officers qualified to administer this type of work and to educate the masses to its needs.

Prevention by eradication

Another disease frequently encountered among school children is trachoma, the destructive importance of which has not yet been generally appreciated. It is a disease of the eyelid which was given to us by a certain class of our foreign immigrants in exchange for liberty and protection. The countries bordering on the Mediterranean and the Orient are the chief contributors, consequently the disease in America is most

Trachoma and its prevention

prevalent at ports of entry where immigration from these countries is heaviest. But the disease is spreading rapidly, especially in schools. It is safe to say that a case infected with trachoma entering school will very soon infect every pupil in attendance if proper preventive measures are not taken. Prevention of this result is within the power of intelligent (medical) school officers and properly educated school teachers and school nurses.

The preceding considerations have dealt largely with questions of epidemics or infectious diseases or with diseases of the indi**Diseases due to social causes** vidual. There is also a large class of humanity which is suffering from disease and disability resulting from social evils, the control of which lies, not only in the hands of the physician, but in the hands of the economist, the clergyman, and the legislator as well. Of these four professions, however, the medical is the one which is brought most closely into contact with the evils of body and mind resulting, and, therefore the physician will always have more closely at heart the alleviation of these sufferings and will enter the field with possibly a more practical idea of methods of relief. Such a man, however, becomes more than a physician, rather a sanitarian in the larger sense—an administrator of State or national health. It is this type of man especially who is to be thought of in the future conduct of a school of preventive medicine. Within **Principles of relief** his realm come not only the administration of problems of public water and food supply, or the health of armies, if his training happen to be in that direction, but also the problems of preventable accidents or dangerous occupations, of school and tenement house conditions, of insanity, of alcoholism, and of poverty dependent upon sickness. It is in preparation for this class of work that a thorough training in economics and social science, finance and jurisprudence, is most important.

The great loss of life resulting from the engagements of warring armies is something to which the nations of the world have **Preventable accidents** partially accustomed themselves, and which they condone in view of centuries of precedent. But few realize or can contemplate with equanimity the fact that of the 29,000,000 workers in these United States in time of peace, more than 500,000 men, women and children, yearly, are killed or crippled as a direct result of the occupations in which they are engaged—more than were slain and wounded throughout the terrible Russo-Japanese war (19). That which renders it appalling is the fact that this is nearly twice the number who meet similar deaths in Europe, and that more than one-half of this tremendous sacrifice of life is needless.

There is no other nation comparable industrially to the United States, which is so backward as this country in its knowledge, in **Dangerous occupations** its legislation, and in its administrative machinery for dealing with the insanitary conditions in factories, mines, and workshops, and in preventing or regulating those dangerous processes in industry that are responsible for a very large number of unnecessary diseases, accidents, and deaths. It is perhaps needless to repeat that these insanitary conditions of home and factory have a direct bearing on the extent of disease and poverty. The field is one which offers the greatest opportunity for humane and merciful legislation. The workmen who are crushed, crippled, or killed, who contract incurable diseases, who are poisoned, or who are incapacitated by carelessness, insanitary conditions, or dangerous machinery, are so numerous in this day that in a very few decades we shall look back upon this period as one of downright barbarism.

That these problems of preventive medicine, falling within the scope of industrial hygiene, are of immense economic importance, **Economic loss from preventable accidents** has been shown by George E. McNeill, President of the International Underwriters Association of America, who estimates the volume of the loss to the country from preventable accident as $348,000,000 a year—equalling one-third the volume of our entire foreign trade. This problem is distinctly an educational one, and its solution must rest with those sanitary administrators who have intimate knowledge of the existing faulty conditions, and upon whose judgment and experience those who are concerned in legislation can rely.

The necessity for intelligence and knowledge of sanitary conditions in the administration of the affairs of tenement house com-

Tenement house sanitation

missions is perhaps nowhere more plainly shown than by reference to an incident which occurred a few years ago in Glasgow, where a frightful death-rate existed among the inhabitants of tenement houses of a certain district (2). The municipal authorities, after becoming acquainted with the conditions, demolished the houses in that section, and built new tenements to take their places. By this act the death-rate was reduced from 55 per thousand to a little over 14 per thousand. An adjoining slum still had a death-rate of 53 per thousand. Here were two groups of houses, sheltering practically the same classes of people, one with a death-rate a little over 14 per thousand, the other with a death-rate nearly four times as great. As an example of the efficacy of intelligent and energetic administration by an officer of health trained in the precepts of public sanitation and prevention, this lesson speaks for itself.

The importance of the relation of disease to poverty, crime, and insanity, is a subject which in the past has been agitated to far

Disease and poverty

too slight an extent. When it is considered that these three conditions, with the immense burdens which they impose upon the state, are due, in part, not only to disease but to preventable disease, the problem opens out into one of intense interest and immense economic importance. While sickness is the source of much pain and of much else that racks the poor old body of humanity, it forces upon thousands and thousands of struggling families an almost greater misery—poverty. No one knows how many thousand families of workingmen, through this cause alone, are brought to distressing poverty and even to miserable pauperism. The charitable organizations say that about one-fourth of the distress which manifests itself is caused by sickness (2). Physical defect prepares the way for dependence on the community, and sickness is a constantly recurring plea of the needy. The bread-winner is incapacitated, the spirit and hope of the family are broken down, and solicitation of help grows into a parasitic habit. The almshouses, asylums and hospitals are crowded with evidences of the close connection between physical infirmity and dependence. The place to strike at this evil is the root, and the most effective method of completing its destruction is by its prevention.

The question whether insanity is increasing faster than population, is one upon which there is a difference of opinion; but the evidence, I believe, leans strongly in favor of the relative increase. For a long time it has been apparent that the number of the insane was everywhere rapidly increasing, that hospitals for the insane were crowded, and that large new establishments were frequently being erected. The 18th Annual Report of the New York State Commission in Lunacy places the number in institutions for the insane in this State at 28,302, of whom 960 were insane criminals. The net increase for the year was 895. The whole number of new cases developing during the year was 5,761. The support of this class of unfortunates and the management of institutions for their care are becoming very burdensome, and to all appearances are likely to become still more so. The State appropriated in 1906 for maintenance, new buildings and for extraordinary repairs to the existing plants, the total valuation of which is $26,000,000, the sum of $5,916,881.83, and the total disbursement for the year for all purposes was $5,722,459.22.

Prevalence of insanity

The impression is becoming general that the multiplication of lunatic hospitals is doing but little to check insanity, and that, if the evil is ever to be checked, some different means must be provided. The more we see of mental disease in its various forms, the more convinced we are that the study of its *prevention* is infinitely more important than even the study of its *cure*. Lunatic hospitals do not prevent insanity because they do not by the intercourse of their officers with society at large, by their published reports, or by their general relations to the public, seek to enlighten the people on the subject of insanity—its predisposing causes, its hereditary tendencies, its relations to syphilis, intemperance, poverty and crime—and therefore they do not improve the community in this respect, except in removing from its care some of its greatest burdens. Ninety per cent. of all the inmates of insane asylums are incurable, hence the rapid increase of chronic insanity which exists (20). What a

Importance of prevention

powerful argument does this fact present in favor of using all possible means for the prevention of the malady!

For the prevention of insanity, then, the same course must be pursued as in preventing other diseases: Ascertain its causes, diffuse information on the subject. This may be accomplished by educational training, through journals and books, by enlisting the press, by legislation and associated action. For illustration: If intemperance and syphilis are the leading causes of insanity, it is high time that the fact should be generally known, and the warning brought home to all. If ill health is adjudged a fruitful source of the malady, let us understand that. If hereditary influences, in all their diversified forms, constitute another fruitful source, let us study better the laws that regulate these influences; or, if fast living or high pressure in our business world or educational systems are steadily swelling the ranks of the insane, the sooner these truths are brought home to the public, the better.

Of all the questions with which the physician has to deal affecting the health, morality and welfare of this country's inhabitants, **Alcoholism** none compares in importance with that pertaining to the use of alcohol as a beverage. The universality of this habit, its far reaching destructive effects, and the burdens which it imposes on the state, render this a problem demanding our best efforts for its solution. The burden of this responsibility has in the past been shouldered by the socialist, the sensationalist, and the politician; but careful analysis of its fundamental problems and causes will readily lead to the conclusion that it is upon the physician—the exponent of state medicine—that the responsibility for the repression of the evil of this habit rests.

The number of habitual drunkards is very much larger than is generally supposed, very many cases of vice being so sheltered **Prevalence of alcoholism** by family life as to escape inclusion in public statistics. It has been estimated that 365,000 men are arrested annually in this country for drunkenness alone— a number larger than that for all other offenses (1). The number of drunkards is not only exceedingly large, but it is increasing, apparently, out of proportion to the increase of population. The physical and mental condition of the habitual drunkard is one of sad deterioration and is replete with misery. His vitality is so lowered that he readily succumbs to any acute disease which may attack him, and upon the occasion of an epidemic, drunkards usually constitute the greater number of those first mown by the scythe of the pestilence. The mind becomes debased; the moral tone, the will and the intellect progressively diminish in power; and alcoholic insanity is the frequent consequence, appearing in the form of melancholia, mania, chronic delirium or dementia—complete obliteration of mental power.

Out of 1,836 cases of insanity, this being the total number found in the institutions of Massachusetts canvassed during twelve **Alcohol and insanity** consecutive months, there were found 671 instances, or 36.55 per cent., in which the person was addicted to the use of liquor. The excessive drinkers numbered 16.94 per cent. of all the insane. The habits of 26.58 per cent. could not be ascertained. Excluding all the minors, whether total abstainers or not, and also excluding the adults about whom the facts as to the use of liquor could not be ascertained, there were 1,281 persons, of whom 51.44 per cent. were addicted to the use of liquor—25 per cent. drinking to excess. Of the cases in which the facts could be ascertained, one or both parents were intemperate in 68.67 per cent. In 20.86 per cent. intemperance was the direct cause of the insanity (21).

The influence of alcohol in the production of diseases other than those of the mind is a far-reaching one. Enumeration of these **Alcohol and disease** in full would be a prodigious task, but in brief the statement is justified that of any one cause alcohol is the most productive of disease. The most common of its effects, apart from those already enumerated, are those seen in peripheral neuritis, Bright's disease and heart disease, cirrhosis of the liver, inflammation of the stomach, and arteriosclerosis, the latter one of the most common causes of apoplexy.

The influence of alcohol on poverty is a matter of no uncertain moment. Boies estimates that alcohol is the direct or indirect **Alcohol and poverty** cause of 50 per cent. of all the suffering endured on account of poverty. On an average, the poverty which comes under the notice of the charity organization societies can be traced to liquor in some 25 per cent. of all the cases, and in almshouses the percentage is 37 (22). The Massachusetts Bureau of Labor (21) reported in 1895, that in that State out of 3,230 paupers, this being the total number found in the State institutions during twelve consecutive months, 2,108, or 65.26 per cent. were addicted to the use of liquor; and 15.63 per cent. of all the paupers used liquor to excess. Of the 2,752 adult paupers, 75.47 per cent. were addicted to the use of liquor, of whom 25 per cent. were excessive drinkers. Of the whole number of paupers, 47.74 per cent. had one or both parents intemperate. Nearly 45 per cent. of the children harbored by humane and orphan asylums owe their destitution to the intemperance of parents (22).

More prolific than any other in the production of crime is the vice of intemperance. This operates in so many ways that it is impossible to trace out all its pernicious effects.

Alcohol and crime

It impoverishes people and brings them into circumstances of temptation; it corrupts the morals and poisons the blood; it excites the evil propensities and develops the animal nature; it stupefies conscience and destroys the moral sentiments; it impairs in man the powers of free agency and converts him into a brute. Whatever produces such effects upon the human system must have a powerful influence in the production of crime. The evidences come from all quarters (and without contradiction from any), that intemperance is the cause or occasion of three-fourths of all the crime committed—some estimating it even higher (20).

If we look at criminal statistics for the effects of this appetite for alcohol, we will find that in the New York City prisons, during 1870, there were out of 49,423 criminals, 30,507 of confessedly intemperate habits. In the Albany Penitentiary there were, in 1869–70, 1,093 convicts, of whom 893 admitted that they were intemperate (23). In France, the average consumption of wine, estimated at 62 liters per head in 1829, exceeded 100 liters in 1869. The total manufacture of alcohol in France (95 per cent. of which is consumed in the form of drink) arose from 479,680 hectoliters in 1843 to 2,004,000 in 1887. Simultaneously there was an increase of crimes and offenses in France, suicides in particular having increased from 1,542 in 1829, to 8,202 in 1887 (24).

Out of 26,672 convictions for various offenses in Massachusetts, during twelve consecutive months, 65.89 per cent. were convictions for drunkenness alone, and 68.36 for drunkenness accompanying some other offense. In 21,863 cases, or 81.97 per cent., the offender was in liquor at the time the offense was committed. Of the whole number of convictions, namely 26,672, the number of offenders addicted to the use of liquor was 25,137 or 94.24 per cent., the excessive drinkers numbering about 16.93 per cent. Of the 25,360 adult offenders, 96 per cent. were addicted to the use of liquor, 17.6 were excessive drinkers. Of the whole number of offenders, 57.89 per cent. had fathers who were addicted to the use of liquor, while 20.49 per cent. had mothers addicted to the use of liquor (21). While, according to Rylands, poverty is considered to be the cause of crime in only 5 per cent. of the cases, intemperance, according to the findings of the Committee of Fifty in its investigations on the liquor problem, figured as one of the causes of crime in New York in nearly 50 per cent. of 13,400 convicts examined (22 and 25).

The expense borne by the State of New York in 1904 for the maintenance of public institutions for the care of these persons was as follows (26):

1. State institutions	$1,796,222.48
2. County Almshouses	1,550,079.57
3. City and Town Almshouse institutions	2,138,288.70
4. Homes for the Blind and Feeble-minded (included in 1 and 2)	
5. Hospitals receiving State aid	5,763,637.33
6. Hospitals and Homes for Consumptives	200,234.94
7. Hospitals and Homes for Epileptics	67,028.03

The total cost to the State alone for the care of the conditions previously cited amounts to $11,515,419 annually. This is far exceeded by the outlay by private charitable institutions for these same purposes, the latter figures, however, being difficult to obtain accurately.

While the diseases thus far mentioned, which we are able and wish to prevent, do not at present all occur in New York City, the list which confronts us is a sufficiently large one to make our task one of no mean proportions.

The problem awaiting solution in New York City at the present time is briefly as follows (8): In 1906, 3,467 people suffered from **The problem of the present day in New York** and 639 died of typhoid fever; and 6,000 died of diarrhœal diseases in Greater New York City, although this could have been almost entirely prevented by a pure water and milk supply: 20,085 suffered from and 10,194 died of tuberculous diseases, although tuberculosis is preventable through the agencies of pure milk supply, personal hygiene, and proper methods of isolation; 164 died of malaria, although this can be prevented by extermination of the mosquito by destroying its breeding places; 36,653 people suffered from and 1,145 died of measles; 7,881 suffered from and 491 died of scarlet fever; 14,757 suffered from and 189 died of diphtheria and croup; 241 died of influenza; 100 suffered from and 6 died of small-pox; 812 died of epidemic cerebrospinal meningitis; 10,868 died of pneumonia; although these diseases are all preventable to a large extent through agencies of personal hygiene, isolation, and modern laboratory methods. Five thousand five hundred and fifty-seven died of heart disease, 6,108 died of nephritis and Bright's disease, and 1,031 died of cirrhosis of the liver—results which could have been diminished through our knowledge already existing of the causes (dietetic, etc.) of these diseases, and may be still more largely diminished by further study into the nature of their causes. Three thousand seven hundred and eighty-one deaths occurred as the result of accident, many of which were preventable by the use of suitable safety devices; and, finally, 3,005 deaths occurred from malignant growth (cancer, etc.) and while not at the present time preventable, the extent of the occurrence of this disease calls for great effort toward obtaining a knowledge of its cause and method of prevention.

The following chart, while illustrating the wonderful decrease in the mortality in New York since 1866, still shows a death-rate of 18.35 per 1,000 population, or about 78,000 deaths a year in Greater New York.

There are 25,000 people in the United States who are needlessly **Preventable blindness** blind, who could have had their vision saved had the causes of blindness and methods for its prevention been widely enough appreciated by the public and the medical profession.

There are 28,302 insane people in New York State under State care, a large number of whom could have escaped insanity had a proper knowledge of the causes of the malady been disseminated among the people, while thousands of cases of disease, crime and poverty occur annually as the result of alcoholism, which could be prevented by diminishing the use of alcohol as a beverage.

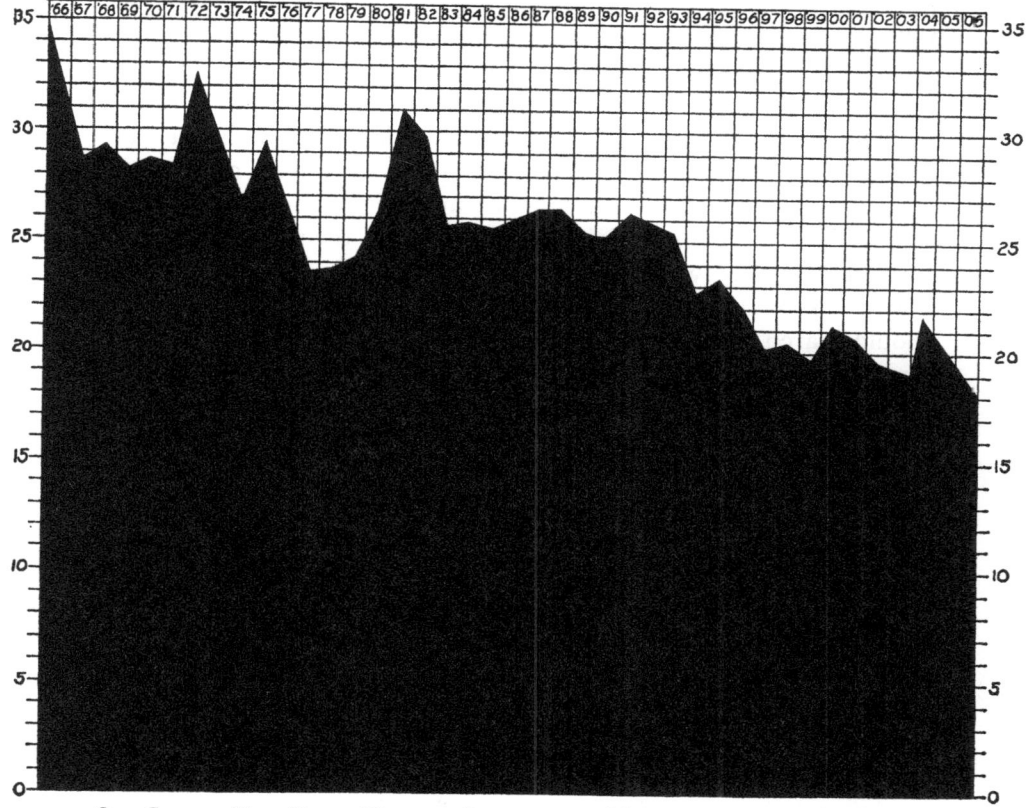

Old City of New York (Present Boroughs of Manhattan and the Bronx)
General Death-Rate Per 1,000 Population. 1866–1906
Courtesy of New York Board of Health

Needlessness of this sacrifice Last year in New York about 30,000 persons died from preventable causes. The time has passed when we can attribute such deaths to the act of Providence. Japan has given the world a tremendously convincing demonstration of how many lives can be bought by money spent for prevention. The facts are well known, but can not be too often repeated. In the recent war with Russia, the Japanese by their elaborate and enlightened educational work, reduced the ratio of deaths due to disease, as compared with those killed in battle, to 1 to 4. In the best managed campaign preceding this, the number of soldiers who died of disease was approximately four times those killed in battle. In our own war with Spain, when there was little attempt to prevent disease and the medical corps was demoralized, the ratio reached the appalling figure of 14 to 1.

The Japanese method cost money. It involved paying a staff of trained medical officers of the same rank as officers of the line, **The Japanese method** and with supreme authority on all sanitary and hygienic questions. With their test-tubes and microscopes they went in advance of the army and determined where it should camp, what waters it should drink, which soldiers should march, and which should go to the hospital. The method likewise saved money. If the same mortality from disease had prevailed in this war as in our own, 840,000 men would have died, and at least 1,680,000 more would have been needed to carry on the struggle. This would have involved the country in utter financial ruin.

The Japanese accomplished this result by careful education of its army and navy officers in principles of sanitation. The need **Needs of our army and navy** for our officers of the army and navy to avail themselves of this training is as great as the present lack of instruction in these lines is apparent. Complete knowledge of this subject can only be obtained by observation of sanitary methods in operation in thickly settled communities, and best obtained by association with a school of preventive medicine.

In summing up, a few statistics will perhaps help the reader to realize that the study of preventive medicine is not a vain one, and **Promise of future relief from past improvement** that the promise of the future is even more brilliant than the results and achievements of the past. Three centuries ago the death-rate of London was more than 80 per 1,000; now it is about 20 per 1,000. It is computed that in the eighteenth century—the one preceding the introduction of vaccination—fifty millions of people died in Europe of small-pox alone; now it is practically almost an extinct disease where vaccination is compulsory, as in Germany. In 1872, Sir John Simon estimated "that the deaths which occur in England are fully a third more numerous than they would be if our existing knowledge of the chief causes of disease were reasonably well applied throughout the country, and that of deaths which in this sense may be called preventable, the yearly average number in England and Wales is about 120,000" (7). In confirmation of the accuracy of this statement, official reports show that the annual death-rate of England and Wales, which averaged 22.6 per 1,000 for the decade of 1862 to 1871, inclusive, fell to 18.9 for 1881, this giving a saving of 92,000 lives annually; while for 1889, even with the correction for the lowered birth-rate, it was only 17.9, indicating a yearly saving of at least 125,000 lives and completely substantiating the above estimate of Simon. Moreover, the death-rate from the seven principal zymotic (infectious) diseases had dropped from an average of 4.11 for the period from 1861 to 1870, to 2.40 for 1881 to 1885, and that for typhoid fever, from 0.39 per 1,000 in 1869, to 0.137 in 1892. This for England and Wales. In Munich, from 1866 to 1881, the average yearly hospital admissions of typhoid fever were 594, or 3.32 per 1,000 of population, and the average deaths from this disease were 208, or 1.15 per 1,000. From 1881 to 1888, following the introduction of improved systems of sewerage and a better water supply, the average hospital admissions (typhoid) were 104, or 0.42 per 1,000, and the average deaths were 40, or 0.16 per 1,000 population.

In this country a like improvement is to be noted, though it is only within the last few decades that much attention has been given to sanitary affairs. The death-rate of most of our cities is being progressively lowered, though the populations are constantly increased by large numbers of ignorant and uncleanly immigrants. Improved sanitary laws are being enacted and enforced; streets are better paved and cared for; more attention is given to isolating the sick and protecting the well, and the people in general are awakening to the importance of improving as well as maintaining the public health. New York City has reduced her death-rate per thousand within the last census decade (1890 to 1900) from 25.4 to 20.5; Chicago, from 19.1 to 16.2; Boston, from 23.4 to 20.1, etc.* (27).

The foundation upon which any institution of preventive medicine must be based rests upon the field of public hygiene, which is that branch of social science which concerns the physical condition of communities. It embraces a consideration of the various influences operating upon society, whether for its material good or its actual deterioration, with the view of extending the former, and preventing or ameliorating, as far as possible, the effects of the latter. It involves the enactment of laws by which the safety of the whole may be protected against the errors of a part; and, above all, it aims at the prevention of disease by the removal of its avoidable causes. In a wide sense, therefore, the science of public hygiene enlists the services of the people in continuous efforts at self-improvement; of the teachers of the people, to inculcate the best rules of life and action; of physicians, to prevent as well as cure disease; and of lawgivers, to legalize and enforce measures of health-preservation.

Principles of prevention and public hygiene

Public health problems, formulated by medical, biological, and scientific evidence, involve legislative, administrative, and social changes of the widest extent in their solution. The social element is a factor to be largely reckoned with. State remedies cannot be applied in advance of public opinion, and this is slow to move. The education of a vast community is perhaps the most difficult task that falls to the sanitarians. Persuading the unscientific mind to reason logically, even after possession of the facts, is not a light task. To rouse it to take action even when convinced, and to overcome prejudice, requires a prodigious effort; *but the task is well worth while.* An idea of the tremendous possibilities of activity in this field may be gathered from the following citations as examples:

Appeal to the public

In the summer of 1906, the Association for Improving the Condition of the Poor inserted articles in the New York papers calling attention to the necessity for increased measures to assure a clean milk supply. As di-

Popular aid in reform

---

* The importance of such statistics is not fully appreciated unless the reader remembers that in a city of, say, a million inhabitants, a reduction of the death rate one point means the saving of one thousand lives annually.

rect and indirect results of such notices may be mentioned a sympathetic hearing on the part of the mayor and the controller, an appropriation enabling the Health Department to double its staff of milk inspectors, an enthusiastic campaign by the *Evening World* that helped to bring about a marked reduction in infant mortality and removed what little doubt had ever existed as to the practicability of securing a clean milk supply and of soon reducing the preventable death-list of babies in the summer from 5,000 to 1,000. Early in July, 1906, the *Evening World* and the Association for Improving the Condition of the Poor began a crusade for "clean air, clean food, and clean babies." July and August, the deadly months for summer-sick little children, saw columns of each day's paper devoted to simple instruction and illustrated talks on the proper care of infants.

In connection with this activity on the part of the press, the following table is of intense interest. It shows strikingly the low rate of mortality in July and early August, 1906, compared with the same period in 1905. This difference is ascribed, to some extent, to this active press campaign of education of the East Side mothers (28).

Relief through activity of press

Owing to the widespread interest aroused by the publication of the facts relating to the physical defects of school children, and to a hearing before the Board of Estimate and Apportionment, $250,850 was voted for medical inspection and examination for the school year 1906–1907. This has made possible the examination of all children in the Borough of Manhattan. The money saved by enabling thousands of children to do one year's work in one year, instead of in two or three years, would greatly exceed the total expense of examining all school children in all boroughs (28). These citations show what far-reaching results can be accomplished by the intelligent direction of efforts along the lines of publicity and press cooperation. It is a modern science created to cope with modern conditions and capable of immense development. This development can be best accomplished in the hands of educators, especially those operating in a central institution for the prevention of the noxious conditions calling forth the effort.

Relief through publicity

These methods of publicity, however, are merely the more popular methods of producing an educational effect which must be

Education and prevention

further extended in more conservative and comprehensive form. It is true that every effort must be made toward the education of the masses as the real

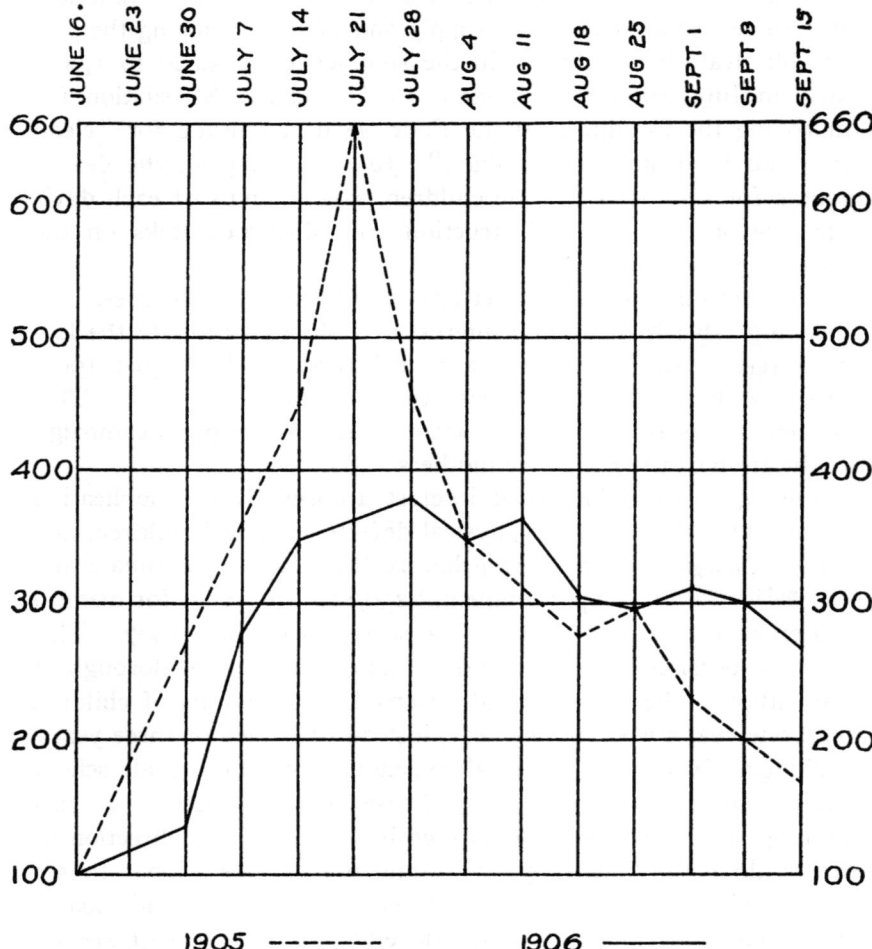

DEATHS OF CHILDREN UNDER FIVE YEARS FROM DIARRHŒAL DISEASES—1905–1906 NEW YORK CITY. Note: The chart is based on the absolute number of deaths, not corrected for increase of population

Courtesy of Association for Improving the Condition of the Poor

groundwork of national health; that the people must be interested systematically in the general policy of prevention, and thus become more intimately acquainted with the social and material causes by which sanitary progress is impeded. But increasing effort must be made to create centers in the form of agents versed in the principles of sanitation, to diffuse this knowledge and aid in insuring its arrival at its ultimate desired goal—the ignorant individual and the filthy home. To this end the desired knowledge of preventive sanitary science should be inculcated in the minds of the future teachers of our public elementary and secondary schools. These teachers have much of the physical as well as the mental welfare of thousands of young and growing children in their keeping, and it is unquestionably their duty to prevent or obviate the ills of school life as far as lies in their power, and to give instruction in, and to inculcate, habits of living which will continually tend to preserve and improve the physical health of those in their care.

At the present time in New York a prodigious effort is being made to improve the condition of the poor by enlisting the services of "social workers" drawn from the better classes of our citizens. If their effort were as well and intelligently directed as their zeal is great, enormous results could be accomplished. The efficiency of their work is considerably enhanced by attendance at an admirably conducted school of philanthropy already existing, but could be still more increased were it possible for them, in wrestling with the daily conditions of imperfect sanitation, to avail themselves of the aid given by a school of preventive medicine.

"Social workers"

Even a still greater result has been and will continue to be accomplished by the powerful educational effect arising from the continuous work of a large body of thoroughly trained health officers and sanitary authorities. As an example of this may be cited the methods employed by the New York Department of Health, under the supervision of Dr. Herman M. Biggs. The Health Department issues from time to time circulars of information on various topics, which are designed for general distribution, particularly among the tenement house population, including such subjects as "Information for con-

Education and health officers

sumptives and their families," "Infant feeding," and "Methods of transmission of contagious diseases." From the bacteriological laboratories numerous scientific bulletins are issued from time to time, detailing the results of original investigations in connection with infectious diseases, and these bulletins are widely distributed among the medical profession of New York City. The importance of this educational work can not be overestimated. Its value is incalculable in widely disseminating popular and scientific information with regard to the results of the latest studies in infectious diseases, and there have been constantly exhibited in New York the most gratifying indications of the influence of the information thus distributed, on both the general public and the medical profession.

Probably the greatest function of a school of preventive medicine would be to train future health officers in methods of administering their positions properly. As an epidemic always falls upon the poor with the greatest violence, and as it is from the poor that most of our infectious diseases spread to the other classes, **Health Boards of the future** it is the duty of the state and to the interest of the other classes, that the health of the poor should be supervised by responsible and capable officials, who know how to perform the work they undertake. It follows, of course, that not only every physician, but every health officer should be well versed in the laws which apply to the prevention of disease and modern sanitary principles. Members of the State boards of health are energetic, intelligent, and progressive in many of the States; but in some no sanitary work of importance is done and, broadly speaking, in the rural districts and in the towns and smaller cities of this country, especially in the south and west, the sanitary methods are of the crudest type (29).

Section 9 of the Act of the Pennsylvania Assembly creating the Health Board, instructs it, "from time to time, to engage **Health Board needs** *suitable persons* to render sanitary service or to make or supervise practical and scientific investigations and examinations requiring *expert skill,* and to prepare plans and reports relative thereto." Observe the phrases "suitable persons" and "expert skill." Heretofore the board has been compelled to call to its aid for these objects simply medical men, intelligent, educated, sound practitioners, but without that special training and equipment which would render them "suitable persons" in any strict, technical construction of the term, or would furnish them with "expert skill." To meet this need a school of preventive medicine is well fitted and would supply a long felt want of all boards of health.

In England, before 1892, the officers of health were usually local practitioners, appointed, not on account of their knowledge of the principles of public health, but on account of their "pull," or in expectation that they would cause less disturbance and accept lower salaries than men who had fully qualified themselves to hold such a post. On and after January 1, 1892, this was markedly changed. In any country district, or combination of districts, having a population of over 50,000, no one could be appointed medical officer of health unless he were a full graduate of medicine and registered as a holder of a diploma from some university body giving instruction in sanitary science, public health or state medicine. This act demanded special training and created a trained body of medical state officers (30).

Fitness for Health Board offices

In this country the efficiency of the administration of our public health service can be best assured only by a demand on the part of the State that its medical officers shall have had the full special training requisite for the performance of their particular duties. It should, therefore, and ultimately will be made obligatory that no one shall be appointed medical officer of health who can not present a diploma from some recognized teaching body, showing that he has passed a satisfactory examination, written and practical, in the subjects of public health and State medicine. By this means the mere political opportunist is barred out from the public health service, as he should be.

But before such a condition can be enforced, facilities for the training of such men must be in operation. The school of preventive medicine would create the material to supply this demand. But there is a still larger scope for the practice of the principles of preventive medicine which is daily assuming a more important aspect in our national life. Conflict between State boards of health as to questions of sanitation that concern the safety of the nation at large is possible, and would be highly detrimental to the public in times of emergency. In times of epidemics it has been very evident that the safety of the nation requires a uniformity and promptness of action incompatible with the independent and often conflicting interests of widely distant State boards. This is particularly the case in a country such as the United States, to whose shores several hundred thousand immigrants come every year, bringing with them, owing to their ignorance and filthy condition, numerous possibilities of disease, unless stringent measures of defense as exemplified in a vigorous quarantine be employed.

These occasions have given rise to the opinion that some national system of supervision of the sanitary condition of the country **National Board of Health** should be introduced here as it has been abroad which, without doing away with State authority should be free to render advice and assistance to the country at large in times of emergency, and should at all times be a medium of communication between different States for diffusing sanitary knowledge and stimulating local sanitation. Such a condition would be fulfilled by the establishment of a national board of health, which would be an agency producing the greatest efficiency in the maintenance of the public health. To fill the positions which the establishment of such a national board would create, there would be the greatest need for sanitarians well trained in schools of public sanitation and preventive medicine, possessing knowledge enabling them to administer the work of departments controlling national quarantine, immigration, sanitation of cities, hygiene of schools and public institutions, infant hygiene, pure food, public water and milk supplies, and statistical and research problems.

A school of preventive medicine should be located in a great city in order that its students, drawn from this class of health **School of Preventive Medicine in a great city** officers, as well as physicians, school teachers, and nurses, social workers, theological students and legislators, may be able to study at first hand such questions as school and tenement house hygiene, dangerous occupations, slaughter houses, water works, and sewage disposal, public nuisances, and compulsory sanitary methods. In such a city as New York, mutual advantage might be secured by such a school, on one hand, and charitable societies for the improvement of social conditions on the other, in aiding each other with training and material. Such an institution should be in the immediate vicinity of and closely connected with a prominent medical school and well-equipped hospitals. Its association with a great university would be of immense value, as by such association it would be enabled to use existing departments of economics and social science, finance, law, education, bacteriology, pathology, medicine, and engineering, already in operation in the parent institution.

Hospital, medical school, and university connections

A factor of great utility in the furtherance of sanitary knowledge in a practical way is one which is employed by the British Sanitary Institute in London. This consists of a museum of sanitation containing all known devices for preventing disease and accident and for improving sanitary conditions, and containing as well those devices which are dangerous to health. It consists of exhibits relating to water supply and sewage, street cleaning, building materials, construction and machinery, articles of personal and domestic hygiene, heating, lighting, and ventilation, and hygiene of special classes, trades and professions relating to schools, trades, hospitals, prisons, barracks, camps, and ships, and the prevention of accidents. This museum is widely utilized, as shown by the annual report of the Council, which gives a list of fifty-two London schools and institutions which send students there for inspection of the exhibits.

Sanitary museum

Valuable training can be given the students of a school of preventive medicine by visits of inspection to public slaughter houses, water supply and sewage disposal works already referred to, disinfecting stations, dairies, factories, and tenements. An added benefit to be derived from this method of class inspection would be the publicity resulting from these visits, as well as the consequent stimulus it would exert toward maintaining these institutions in their most sanitary and effective condition.

Inspection classes

The instruction of the teachers and the health protectors of the public is a most important function of a school of preventive medicine. There is a further most urgent need, however, in the capacity of advisory council constituted to judge the merits of debatable preventive measures, illustrated, for example, by the following: The tendency to postpone the benefits of new medical discoveries bids fair in the future to rival that of the past. The delay in such matters as the application of antitoxins, of the proper treatment of tuberculosis, and the best methods for milk and water purification, has cost thousand of lives and should be obviated. Such an institution, then, should assume the functions of a court of investigation and procedure, which, investigating the efficiency of methods already known and having the confidence of the public, could decide intelligently and without delay, problems that, in our present chaotic state of indecision, are allowed to remain *sub judice* for far too long a time.

Court of appeal

It has been true for decades, not only that the application of beneficial methods in medicine has been very slow, but that very frequently the application of scientific discoveries has been difficult to secure on account of popular ignorance and legislative bias and inertia. Even such a valuable scientific discovery as vaccination against small-pox is of very little use in exterminating this preventable disease until its general application is secured through the agency of popular and legislative action.

Relation of law to sanitary advance

The extent of information available at the present time for improving the conditions under consideration would be sufficient, if properly applied, to cause the effacement of a large proportion of the miseries of mankind. But this information is not now so applied and it remains for an educational body of this kind to correlate it and so bring it within the grasp of those able to profit by its application, that the benefits to be obtained by the full utilization of this knowledge may be enjoyed.

Existing knowledge sufficient if applied

And, finally, it would be the function of such a school to maintain fellowships, the possessors of which, scholars of ability, should inquire into the methods of diminishing human suffering, the result of social conditions and of causes not well known. These workers would make a study of

Research

statistics and conditions bearing on disease and social problems at home and abroad, deriving their knowledge from the scientific triumphs of the present day and the experience of the past.

After man's patient waiting through the centuries, the day has at last arrived when, the instruments having been placed in his hands, he is able to drive back suffering and desolation. The doors have been opened admitting light and knowledge into the remotest depths of pestilential abysses. For centuries man was compelled to bear the chagrin of feeling that all the devastation and destruction of life were from causes beyond his understanding, and the sacrifice one which achieved little in teaching him how to obviate these miseries. But relief has arrived and is now in the possession of those of us who, utilizing our resources to these ends, will avail ourselves of those weapons placed so opportunely in our hands to further our cause and apply the lesson derived from the world's great sacrifice.

Time ripe for advance

Benefit from past sacrifice

When we look around us and consider the condition of the world: the abundance of life, its appalling waste; the wonderful contrivances of the animal kingdom, the apparent indifference with which they are trampled under foot; the gift of mind, its awful perversions and alienations; and when, especially, we note the condition of the human race, and consider what it apparently might be, and what it is: its marvelous endowments and lofty powers, its terrible sufferings and abasements; its capacity for happiness, and its cup of sorrow; the boon of glowing health, and the thousand diseases and painful deaths—that soul must indeed be lethargic and callous which does not glow with an overpowering desire to elevate the good and annihilate the misery, and, utilizing our knowledge of the cause of all this sorrow for its further prevention, resolve that all these dead and suffering shall not have died and suffered in vain.

The improvement in the condition of mankind during the past century has been such that its contemplation will always be the source of supreme gratification to the human race; but, great as has been the progress in the

Possibilities of the future

past, the possibilities of the future almost exceed the realms of most sanguine anticipation.

> "The new
> Shall do
> The unknown things, the wondrous deeds,
> Earth's future needs
> Demand;
> Its hand
> Shall shape the course
> Its brain devise the plan
> to win the richest prize that man can win—
> The betterment of man."

It is blessed to relieve human miseries; it is still more blessed to prevent them.

NEW YORK, March 1, 1907.

APPENDIX I

SCOPE OF A SCHOOL OF PREVENTIVE MEDICINE. METHODS AND COURSE OF STUDY

A school of preventive medicine should be planned to give instruction to the following groups:

1. Students preparing for the practice of medicine.
2. Students preparing for offices of health boards and sanitary inspectors.
3. Students preparing for sanitary engineering—civil, military and naval.
4. Students preparing for work as school and college teachers, school nurses and school inspectors.
5. Students preparing for work as officers of charity societies and institutions, visiting nurses and "social workers."
6. Students preparing for the ministry.
7. Students preparing for the work of legislators.
8. The public.

The following subjects should be taught to the groups designated:

Education and Preventive Medicine

	Physicians	Health Officers	Sanitary Engineers	School Teachers	School Nurses	School Inspectors	Theological Students	Legislators	Charity Society Officers	"Social Workers"
Conditions concerned in the causation and occurrence of disease in individuals, groups of individuals, and communities	+	+	+	+	+				+	+
Modes of transmission, portals of infection, geographical and seasonal distribution of transmittable and epidemic diseases, and the approved methods of prevention of these and other diseases	+	+	+	+	+	+			+	+
Legal aspects of methods of isolation, quarantine, medical and sanitary inspection, compulsory vaccination and inoculation, school attendance, notification, and of methods for preventing the transmission of communicable and epidemic diseases	+	+	+	+	+	+	+	+	+	+
The liquor problem; insanity, pauperism and crime dependent on disease and intemperance	+	+	+	+	+	+	+	+	+	+
American social conditions (including immigration, the growth and concentration of population in cities, with the attendant dangers)	+	+	+	+	+	+	+	+	+	+
*The labor problem	+						+	+	+	+
Sanitary legislation and organization	+	+	+	+	+	+		+	+	+
*Principles of relief; organized charities	+			+	+		+		+	+
*Communistic and socialistic theories; *Social reform; *Sociology and social evolution; *The standard of living; *Poverty and dependence	+						+	+	+	+
Social and moral prophylaxis	+	+		+	+		+	+	+	+
*Political economy and finance	+	+						+	+	
*Pathological psychology; *Disease of the mind and nervous system	+						+		+	+
Medical and sanitary inspection	+	+	+			+				
Safety appliances and the enforcement of their use	+	+					+	+		+
Diseases of animals transmittible to man; Relation of insects to disease	+	+	+	+	+	+		+	+	+
Army and Naval hygiene	+	+	+				+			
Hygiene of the child and the adult, the school and the tenement house, hygiene of ventilation, heating, atmospheric pollutions, and their influence on health and disease	+	+	+	+	+	+	+	+	+	+
*Theory and practice of physical education	+	+		+	+	+	+		+	+
Sanitary engineering of buildings, including plans and sites for hospitals, schools, tenements, etc.; also drainage, plumbing, ventilation, etc.	+	+	+						+	
Prevention of disease requiring knowledge of engineering problems (as at Panama and in Cuba, etc.), drainage of swamps to prevent malaria, etc.	+	+	+						+	
Municipal, State, and national government	+	+	+	+			+	+		
Medical jurisprudence										

* Course already existing in Columbia University.

	Physicians	Health Officers	Sanitary Engineers	School Teachers	School Nurses	School Inspectors	Theological Students	Legislators	Charity Society Officers	"Social Workers"
Correction of conditions which interfere with the physical welfare of school children..........	+	+	+	+	+	+	+	+	+	+
*Social and vital statistics....................	+	+	+	+	+	+	+	+	+	+
Adulterated and unwholesome food; markets, bakeries, hotels, restaurants, infected food, ice, canned goods and water supplies........	+	+	+	+	+	+	+	+	+	+
Dairy products; Milk, etc.; Inspection of herds and dairies; Use of tuberculin test, pasteurization, milk analysis and laws..............	+	+	+	+	+	+	+	+	+	+
Dangerous occupations and preventable accidents......................................	+	+	+			+		+	+	+
Municipal sanitation: Pollution of water and ice supplies, methods of purification and relation to health and disease............................. Construction of reservoirs, filtration plants, sewage and water systems; Methods of sewage and refuse disposal; Street cleaning Public baths, parks, and comfort stations Public nuisances, offensive trades, smoke, stables, noises and filth................	+	+	+	+				+		+
Laboratory courses in analysis of water, air, milk, food, etc. *Bacteriology, *Pathology, *Chemistry.................................	+	+	+							
Excursions for sick children, fresh air funds, visiting nursing, etc......................	+				+	+	+		+	+
Sanitary museum exhibits (see Parke's Museum catalogue)................................	+	+	+	+	+	+	+	+	+	+
*Domestic Science...........................										

* Course already existing in Columbia University.

The education of the public is to be accomplished through the medical profession, health officers, charity societies, the clergy, labor organization leaders, the press, and by public exhibitions of methods of prevention. (Familiar examples are the Exhibition of the Prevention of Tuberculosis and the Exhibition of Safety Appliances to diminish preventable accidents. Sanitary Museum.)

Through these agencies results are to be produced by instruction in personal hygiene, the value of physical training, methods of transmission of disease, methods of prevention, the liquor question, the insane, the criminal, physical welfare of children, social and moral prophylaxis, the use of organized charities and public institutions, need for legislative action, action by municipal authorities and boards of health.

One of the great duties of an institution of learning is the advancement of knowledge. This is accomplished by means of (*a*) laboratory research, and (*b*) higher research into social and scientific methods.

The first involves research into the causation of those diseases of which the causes are at present only imperfectly known or not at all, and into methods for their prevention. Under this class come especially cancer, diabetes, chronic rheumatism and gout, heart disease and Bright's disease—the last probably being due to conditions of diet and nutrition which urgently demand laboratory investigation of a chemical nature. As observations on these diseases are made to the best advantage on patients in hospitals, this research work should be carried on at a place most convenient to the hospital wards, that is, in hospital laboratories.

In connection with health boards, research might well be devoted to the investigation and preparation of antitoxins, vaccines, etc., for the prevention and cure of disease; also investigation of the efficiency of filtration and disinfection methods.

Fellowships should be founded, the holders of which, by availing themselves of material from boards of health and all known sources, should strive to solve such problems as the following: Relations between varieties of food and disease; results obtained by the use of pasteurized milk, immunization by vaccination and antitoxin administration, seashore and mountain hospitals, etc.; utilization of sewage for commercial purposes; methods of cremation, and disposal of garbage; modes of transmission of contagious diseases; study of epidemics and their causes; best methods for the prevention of alcoholism, preventable accidents, venereal diseases, insanity and social conditions causing disease (child labor, etc.); collection of social and vital statistics for specific purposes; clinics or inspection classes.

Students should be brought face to face with the conditions requiring improvements and shown existing departments pertaining to health problems in action. Such subjects are the following: Tenement houses; offensive trades and dangerous occupations; child labor and factories; sweat shops; slaughter houses, dairies, markets, water sheds; appliances in use to prevent accidents; municipal departments of water supply, sewage and refuse disposal, street cleaning, and health department.

APPENDIX II

BIBLIOGRAPHY

1. The Economics of Disease. McKim.
2. Poverty. Robert Hunter.
3. Results of Municipal Sanitation. M. G. Dana, M.D. *Annals of Hygiene,* 1896, vol. 11, p. 391.
4. A Manual of Hygiene. Bissell.
5. The Bubonic Plague. Walter Wyman. Treasury Department.
6. Text-book of Hygiene. Rohe.
7. Hand Book of Hygiene and Sanitary Science. Wilson.
8. Annual Report of the Department of Health of the City of New York. 1904.
9. Yellow Fever Institute Bulletins Nos. 1, 2, 3, 4, 5, 6 and 7.
10. Walter Reed and Yellow Fever. H. A. Kelly.
11. Hygiene of Transmissible Diseases. Abbott.
12. The New Hygiene. Metchnikoff.
13. The Real Triumph of Japan. Seaman.
14. Preventive Medicine. C. A. Boice.
15. The Possibilities of Modern Medicine. A. C. Seely, M.D. *Leslie's Magazine,* June, 1905.
16. Rabies. M. P. Ravenel, M.D. Penn. Dep't of Agriculture, Bulletin No. 79.
17. Rentoul.
18. Vital Statistics. A. Newsholme.
19. Our Industrial Juggernaut. Arthur B. Reeve. *Everybody's Magazine,* February, 1907.
20. The Prevention of Disease, Insanity, Crime and Pauperism. N. Allen, M.D.
21. 26th Annual Report of the Massachusetts Bureau of Labor. Report on the Statistics of Labor. Massachusetts, 1905.
22. The Liquor Problem. Committee of Fifty.
23. The Dangerous Classes of New York. C. L. Brace.
24. Criminal Sociology. Ferri.
25. Crime: Its Causes and Remedy. Gordon Rylands.
26. 38th Annual Report of the State Board of Charities of the State of New York. 1904.
27. Hygiene and Sanitation. Egbert.
28. 63d Annual Report of the Society for Improving the Condition of the Poor. 1906.
29. Preventive Medicine. Biggs.
30. The Double Allegiance of the Medical Officers of Health. J. G. Adami, M.D., F.R.S.

Principles of Sanitary Science and the Public Health. Sedgwick.
Public Hygiene and Preventive Medicine. Lewis and Balfour.
Practice of Medicine. Osler.
Annual Report of the Michigan State Board of Health. 1896.
The Causes and Prevention of Phthisis. Milroy Lectures. 1890. Arthur Ransome, M.D.
Manual of Hygiene. Hamer.
Dependents, Defectives, Delinquents. Henderson.
Parke's Hygiene.
Preventive Medicine in the City of New York.
Principles of Hygiene. Bergey.
Proposed Sterilization of Certain Mental and Physical Degenerates.
27th Annual Report of the Massachusetts State Board of Charity. 1905.
The Restriction and Prevention of Dangerous Diseases. Henry B. Baker, M.D. *Annals of Hygiene,* 1890, vol. 5, No. 9.
The Prevention of Disease. William W. Potter, M.D. *N. Y. Medical Journal,* 1894, vol. 59, p. 450.
Preventive Medicine. Sir Peter Eade, M.D. *Popular Health Magazine,* 1895, vol. 11, No. 7.
The Objects, Plans and Needs of the Laboratory of Hygiene. John S. Billings, M.D. *Boston Medical and Surgical Journal,* vol. 126, No. 8, p. 181.
Address. B. Lee, M.D. *Boston Medical and Surgical Journal,* vol. 126, No. 8, p. 184.
Address on the Opening of the Institute of Hygiene of the University of Pennsylvania. S. Weir Mitchell, M.D. *University Med. Magazine,* vol. 4, No. 6, p. 401.
Handbook of Practical Hygiene. Bergey.
Preventive Medicine of Public Health. Alfred Carpenter, M.D.
New York Department of Health. Circular of Information Regarding the Causation and Prevention of Cerebro-Spinal Meningitis.
Mortality Statistics in the United States. 1897. Marine Hospital Service.
Yellow Fever in France, Italy, Great Britain and Austria. Yellow Fever Bulletin, No. 8.
Report of Working Party No. 2. Yellow Fever Institute Bulletin, No. 14.
Report of Working Party No. 1. *Ibid.*

Bei Fragen zur Produktsicherheit wenden Sie sich bitte an:
If you have any questions regarding product safety,
please contact:

Walter de Gruyter GmbH
Genthiner Straße 13
10785 Berlin
productsafety@degruyterbrill.com